A Patient's Guide to Stem-Cell Therapy

Dr. Luis G. Romero

Dr. Jorge L. Gaviño

ISBN-13: 978-1-985-890-183
ISBN-10: 1-985-890-186

If you are interested in Stem cell treatments or want to know more about the subject, feel free to contact:

Dr. Luis Romero or Dr. Jorge Gaviño at ProgenCell

Phone: + 1 (888) 443-6235

Email: info@progencell.com

Websites:
www.patientsguidestemcelltherapy.org
www.progencell.com

DEDICATION

To our lovely family. Thank you so much for your patience, support and unconditional love.

To our patients, you are our motivation in life. Without you we wouldn't have any purpose. Thank you to all the patients that have trusted us, putting their health into our hands, searching for hope & getting a solution to their problems. Thank you for challenging us to grow our knowledge in different areas of medicine.

To our team. No one, by himself, can build an organization. Every single member of a team has a big role in every step of growth. The efforts of everyone combined with such passion eventually take the team to the top of the mountain. Thank you very much for your long hours, your support and expertise.

ACKNOWLEDGEMENT

This book is for patients looking to learn about stem cell therapy. Those who do not give up with traditional medicine, and those who like to explore options into the natural perfection of the human body.

We would like to thank our friend Abraham Elias B. and Dr. Kiran K. who helped with ideas, gathering data, translating papers and with the coordination of this work. Without them, this book wouldn't be in your hands.

WARNING AND DISCLAIMER

This book contains research and opinion of the authors. The authors have successfully treated many patients and the information on this book summarizes many years of experience. It is written as an educational piece for patients interested on the subject of general health and its interaction with stem cells. This book has the intent to educate, it is not intended as medical advice and does not replace supervision of a professional doctor for any kind of treatment.

The information on this book may not be suitable for every patient and we do not guarantee it will cure any disease or produce any particular result. The authors and publishers made considerable efforts to ensure the accuracy of the information provided, and disclaim any responsibility for any liability, loss or risk, personal or otherwise, which is incurred as a consequence, directly or indirectly, from the use and application of any of the content of this book and its associated material.

Laws and medical practices often vary from country to country and patients are heavily encouraged to seek professional medical advice prior going into any medical treatment.

TABLE OF CONTENTS

INTRODUCTION

This book is intended for patients' early adopters of technology. Patients that have tried traditional medicine and have not gotten the expected results. Patients tired of swallowing a pill every day, to control one disease but increasing the risk factors on another organ, or getting a secondary effect that is harmful in the long run.

You may know someone with one of these situations, and our purpose is to educate on what we have learned over the years. Even though this book is not intended as a medical advice, it is organized as a guide with the intention to inform any person about what is stem cell therapy. In the first chapters we go through general information to educate people about what are stem cells and how they can be useful for some people. Then we share our experience on specific diseases that we (or someone else) have treated successfully and how are the medical procedures performed. At the end of the book we try to put useful information to the reader such as our expectations of the future of medicine and tips of how to choose a clinic if you ever want to get stem cell therapy.

This book has been written for the benefit of patients. We really hope people do not suffer if something can be done; we do not want to see families traveling all over the world, spending tons of money trying to find miracle cures following misleading information. Patients have enough trouble just getting by over their limitations because of their illness; it is a shame that some fraudulent organizations offer dishonest treatments for financial purposes.

We understand how these patients and their families feel because we see it very often. We get patients very sick after going through many different promising treatments that may have put them in worse shape. Also with a plunged economical situation that could endanger the financial position of even their entire family. When you add up all the factors: medical condition, not being able to work, financial breakdown and family matters, among others, the patient (and close family members) is steering into a bad depression. Very negative thoughts can surface and fall into a bottomless negative spiral.

We like to think that we can help break the negative spiral, reversing the whole situation into a positive spiral. If we can make the patient feel better, he will eat better, have daily activities, then the family can become functional again. Reducing medical expenses and the patient getting productive again are factors that bring happiness not only for the patient but also for the whole family. Since every person's mind is their own world, we can relate to one of our favorite quotes:

"Whoever saves one life, saves the world entire."

Talmud Yerushalmî

1

WHAT ARE STEM CELLS?

There has been a lot of news about stem cells in the recent past as far as advancements in medical therapy are concerned. It has been nearly five decades since stem cell therapy was applied to humans.

The first successful bone marrow transplant was conducted by Robert A. Good of the University of Minnesota on a child patient suffering from an immune deficiency that affected other family members as well. The boy received bone marrow from his sister, and he grew into a healthy adult.

WHAT IS A STEM CELL?

In modest words, a stem cell is the pioneer cell in the body that has the capability to develop into various kinds of body cells (such as blood cells, skin cells, etc.) during early stages of life and growth.[1] Moreover, in numerous tissues they serve as an internal repair framework, isolating basically unbounded to renew different cells until the individual or the creature is still alive. At the point, when the stem cell divides, each new cell has the potential either to remain a stem cell or turn into another kind of cell with a more particular role, for example, a muscle cell, a brain cell, or a blood cell.

A more intricate definition would be that it is an undifferentiated cell of a multicellular organism, which has the ability to give rise to indefinite cells of the same type, and from which other kinds of cells arise by differentiation.

Stem cells are unique among other body cells because they possess the following important characteristics:

- They are unspecified cells: They have the ability to renew themselves by cell division.

- Ability to become specified

- cells: Certain conditions (physiological or experimental) can induce them to divide into more specialized tissue - or organ - specific cells. Such as, in the bone marrow and the GIT, stem cells divide regularly to repair and replace tissues that are damaged. Whereas, in the heart and the pancreas, they can divide only under certain conditions. [2]

The History of Stem Cells

The story of stem cells has a beginning, a middle but no end. Until lately, scientists predominantly worked with embryonic stem cells and adult / somatic stem cells (non-embryonic) derived from humans and animals. These cells will be explained in detail later in this chapter. This groundbreaking discovery in the field of medicinal research has revolutionized the mainstay of cell-based therapy for a wide spectrum of diseases. Here is a timeline that shows the evolution of stem cell research. [3]

1981, BEGINNINGS IN MICE:

More than three and a half decades ago, G R Martin; Evans and Kaufman discovered ways to isolate embryonic stem cell from early embryos of mice.

1997, DOLLY, THE FIRST CLONED SHEEP:

Dolly was the first ever cloned animal. Ian Wilmut and his team fused a sheep egg with an udder cell and then implanted it into a surrogate female sheep.

1998, STEM CELLS WERE GROWN IN THE LABORATORY:

Thomson J and his team derived stem cell lines from human blastocysts (a 3 to 5 days old embryo) based on the detailed study of stem cells of mice. These human blastocysts-derived stem cells are known as "human embryonic stem cells".

2001, POLITICAL CONTROVERSY:

George W. Bush, the then president of the United States had limited the funding/grants for human embryonic stem cell research. He stated that it was unethical because human embryos were destroyed in the process.

2005, FAKE CLONE CONTROVERSY:

There was a lot of buzz about using human embryonic stem cells to clone genes that were specific to certain people. This would open up a whole new realm of safety and unethical issues. Later on, it turned out these claims were false.

2006, CELLS WERE REPROGRAMMED:

Shinya Yamanaka of Kyoto University in Japan made another breakthrough by isolating "induced pluripotent stem cells". He harvested adult stem cells and reprogrammed them under certain circumstances to act like embryonic stem cells. This abolished the need of destroying embryos.

2007, NOBEL PRIZE

By introducing specific modifications in a gene by using embryonic stem cells of mice, Sir Evan JM, Capecchi MR, and Smithies O were jointly awarded the Nobel Prize in the field of Medicine or Physiology.

2009, OBAMA REIGN

With President Obama in office, the restrictions on stem cell research were lifted.

2010, STEM CELL THERAPY WAS APPLIED

A person with a spinal injury received medical treatment with stem cells derived from a human embryo. This was a trial carried out by Geron.

2012, BLINDNESS TREATED:

Stem cell therapy was used to treat blindness. This too was revolutionary.

2013, ANOTHER NOBEL PRIZE:

Yamanaka and John Gurdon were jointly awarded the Nobel Prize for crafting induced pluripotent stem cells. This was the second Nobel Prize awarded for stem cell research.

2014, THERAPEUTIC CLONING:

Shoukhrat Mitalipov and colleagues produced human embryonic stem cells from fetal cells using therapeutic cloning.

WHY ARE STEM CELLS IMPORTANT?

Learning about stem cells is still considered a groundbreaking achievement in the field of science and research. The possibilities we can achieve through stem cell research is unlimited. One of the most important and obvious functions of a stem cell is that it can develop into a human being. This is a fascinating aspect of stem cell research. The evolution of a single unspecialized cell into a million highly specialized cells. This unravels so many questions, but the important one is 'How'? The challenge of answering this question is being toiled upon for so many reasons.

Given their exceptional regenerative capacities, stem cells offer new possibilities for treating certain medical conditions like cardiovascular diseases and diabetes. Nevertheless, there remains much work to be done in the research center and the facility to recognize how to utilize these unique cells as reparative or regenerative medicine comprising cell-based therapies to treat the infection.

Here are a few of the potential outcomes of stem cell research, much more will be discussed in detail throughout the course of the book.

DIABETES:

Type I diabetes is caused by degeneration of insulin-producing cells of the pancreas by the person's own immune system, hence called an 'auto-immune' disease. Research now reveals that stem cells can be regulated and grown in a controlled environment to yield healthy insulin-producing cells. The outcomes, from our experience of working at ProgenCell, with Autologous adult stem cells from bone marrow are:

- Reduced consumption of insulin

- Regulated immune system

- Prevention of further complications

HEART DISEASE:

Heart disease is one of the leading causes of death worldwide. It is a well-known fact that once healthy heart tissue is damaged, it can't be undone. Research has been performed using adult stem cells from a non-heart tissue. When transplanted into a damaged heart, they begin to regenerate healthy heart tissue. However, a direct transplant is still in the experimental phase and has been carried out in mice. Having said this, our results with intravenously infused autologous adult stem cells has been astonishing. It has shown to increase the vascular ejection fraction of cardiac patients as well as reduce the angina pain.

BIRTH DEFECTS:

Stem cell research has unthinkable potential results when it comes to finding out how birth defects occur. Preventive techniques can be sought and may even possibly someday be reversed. A comprehensive understanding of the regulation and chemical stimuli of stem cell multiplication and differentiation is vital to addressing birth defects.

CANCER:

Cell-based therapy/cell-replacement therapy is the

foundation of discovering a cure for cancer. Cancer, be it in any form, is caused by abnormal proliferation of the body's own cells. Sometimes it associated with a gene mutation, sometimes it's not. Using a stem cell which has the potential to replicate in hundreds of naïve cells and tweaking it to defeat the cancer cells is a feat in itself. For instance, certain bone cancers, like leukemia are being treated with bone marrow transplants. It is based on the regenerating principle of stem cells where healthy cells replace the proliferating cancer cells that originate in the bone marrow itself. It is often a lifesaving procedure. [4]

WHAT IS THE NATURE OF A STEM CELL AND HOW DOES IT FUNCTION?

The human body contains many specialized cells, which carry out specific functions. These are called differentiated cells. In contrast, a stem cell is undifferentiated. It gives rise to multiple cell types including more stem cells.

A stem cell is formed when a sperm penetrates an egg. This is a special kind of stem cell, called a zygote and has the potential to grow into a human being. For the first few divisions, all the cells remain undifferentiated. Each cell has the same turnover as the fertilized egg initially, as far as cell type is concerned. As the development phase continues, a series of signals or instructions gradually limit each cell's potential. Differentiation has begun.

WHAT DOES CELL POTENTIAL MEAN?

Generally, the term potential refers to the inherent capability of coming into being, or likely to become or be. When applied to a stem cell, it connotes the inherent ability of a stem cell to:

- Divide and renew itself

- Be unspecialized by nature

- Form specialized cells

This might sound contradicting. How can something which is simple by nature produce something so complex? Well, as a stem cell is dividing or proliferating, there comes a point where special instructions or signals influence the innate nature of that cell. The cell is instructed from the inside as well as from the outside. The inner signals are transmitted by the cell's own genes, while the outer signals are relayed by certain chemicals present in the microenvironment surrounding the cell. Adjacent cells also release certain chemicals which serve as signals for the stem cell. As a result of this sophisticated exchange of information, an ordinary stem cell gives rise to a cell with a specialized function of its own.

This natural exchange of information and signals is still under research in hopes to someday control and regulate the growth of stem cells in a laboratory for research purposes and to refine cell-based therapies in the future.

HOW DO THE CELLS DIFFERENTIATE INTO A HUMAN BEING?

About one week after fertilization the embryo looks like a hollow ball. The cells on the outside of the blastocyst (hollow ball) will form the placenta and the cells lining the inside will form the different parts of the body. The placenta is an organ which connects the fetus to the mother's womb by implanting its roots in the uterine wall. Food and nutrition, travel to the fetus, while excreted toxins flow out from the fetus via the umbilical cord and the placenta.

After about two weeks the inner cell mass organizes into three layers and each cell's potential is further decreased.

1. *Ectoderm* (outer layer) forms the skin, nervous system, and parts of the face and neck.

2. *Mesoderm* (middle layer) forms the muscles, blood, blood vessels, and the beginning of connective tissue.

3. *Endoderm* (inner layer) form the digestive and respiratory tract, and certain glands like the pancreas and liver.

CLASSIFICATION OF STEM CELLS

In order to understand how stem cells function, it is essential to know a bit about different groups, they belong to. There are four basic classifications of stem cells based on their nature, function, origin and potency. [5]

Allogeneic vs Autologous stem cells:

When a stem cell is used for therapy it is very important to discern which body it came from. An allogeneic transplant involves stem cells taken from a donor. An autologous transplant uses the recipient's own stem cells. There are pros and cons for each method, but autologous transplant is seen to have minimal unwanted effects. Allogeneic stem cells have the potential to generate rejection and cause a reaction on the receptor.

Embryonic vs Adult stem cells:

A common classification of stem cells is based on the location of origin. Stem cells derived from an embryo are termed as embryonic stem cells or ESCs (embryo is usually formed in vitro, i.e. outside of a woman's body for research purposes). ESCs are easier to grow in culture (lab) than ASCs.

Adult stem cells (also called somatic stem cells) are undifferentiated stem cells, which reside in a small 'niche' of their own within a differentiated tissue. They have a controlled self-renewal ability. ASCs are found in many organs and tissues like skin, blood vessels, peripheral blood, bone marrow, teeth, skeletal muscle, brain, heart, liver, gut, testis, and, ovarian epithelium.

A significant use of both ESCs and ASCs is their consumption in cell-based therapies. Since an ESC has the ability to differentiate into any type of cell, scientists could manipulate/reprogram its genes to yield a certain type of cell. For instance, a recent research carried out in King's College London was able to derive an embryonic stem cell line that carried a mutation in the SMN1 gene. This gene mutation is associated with a disease known as Spinal Muscular Atrophy. The scientists were able to assess and study the different stages of differentiation. Maybe in the future, they will be able to reprogram the gene mutation in attempts to cure the disease linked to it.

An ASC can be used in the same way. Since they are limited in number and further limited in their differentiation potential, they are preferred for stem cell therapies. Accessing them to such a degree is challenging, but there are concentrated areas in the body where they can be found and collected without major risks or side effects such as umbilical cord blood in newborns and bone marrow in adults.

Besides the difficulty to control ESCs for practical use outside the lab, in many places of the world ESCs are prohibited and illegal due to the controversy that surrounds it. A lot of discussions happen around ethical and religious issues, therefore they are not commonly used for human stem cell therapy.

Stem cell potential:

TOTIPOTENT (OMNIPOTENT) STEM CELLS

A totipotent stem cell has the ability to differentiate into any type of cell in an organism. The best example of a TSC is a 'zygote' (fertilized egg). It can give rise to embryonic as well as extraembryonic tissues. In the initial developmental phase, the zygote keeps dividing to yield more totipotent cells. It is approximately after 4 days that the totipotent cells begin to differentiate or specialize into pluripotent cells. So, what makes a totipotent cell unique? Well, first, it has the ability to form any type of cell in a human being and second, it possesses the capability of producing an unlimited number of cells without losing its total potency. What are the challenges? Controlling their growth and their differentiation is difficult. They behave as wild cells, so trying to control them for human therapy has been a safety challenge.

PLURIPOTENT STEM CELLS

A pluripotent stem cell is also called a 'true stem cell'. As mentioned above, pluripotent stem cells arise from totipotent cells.

The first batch of pluripotent stem cells is seen in the form of an inner cell mass at the blastocyst stage of fetal development. The blastocyst as mentioned above consists of a cluster of cells lining the inside of the blastocyst, which gives rise to the human organs, tracts and glands. These pluripotent cells are able to self-renew and differentiate into either of the three germ layers mentioned above i.e. the ectoderm, mesoderm or endoderm. The germ layers, in turn, form the different components of a human being. [6]

Pluripotent stem cells have a widespread use in the treatment of various diseases and conditions like heart disease, diabetes, burn victims and even neurological disorders like Parkinson's disease. This is only possible due to its inherent property of differentiating into almost any cell type like heart, nerve, muscle, etc. Pluripotent cells have also proved useful in the drug industry, particularly in the drug testing phase. Before being tested on animals, the effects of certain drugs are seen in PSCs. If the cells tolerate the drug without any adverse effects, further testing is moved on to the animals. A close human-made kin of the PSC is an induced PSC. An iPSC can be re-programmed to function as an embryonic stem cell.

INDUCED PLURIPOTENT STEM CELLS

An iPSC is an adult cell created in a lab that has been genetically reprogrammed to mimic an embryonic stem cell by enforcing it to express genes and factors necessary for maintaining the characteristic and properties of embryonic stem cells. The advent of iPSCs has opened up several avenues in the pharmaceutical industry, clinics, and laboratories. In particular, the medical uses of human iPSCs in the modification of disease and stem cell therapy have not been progressing much, still a long way to go. Mostly they have been used in the lab for drug testing. The cell-inducing property is not only attractive for its medical applications, but also for basic cancer research, pharmaceuticals, genetics, and ageing.

MULTIPOTENT STEM CELLS

A multipotent stem cell can give rise to more than one cell type, but is more restricted in its function. A good example would be a mesenchymal stem cell which can develop into bone, muscle and cartilage cells. Other examples include adult stem cells and cord blood stem cells

UNIPOTENT STEM CELL

A unipotent stem cell differentiates along a single lineage of cells. For instance, a muscle cell has the ability to self-renew, but only into a specific type of muscle cell. Out of all the stem cells, it has the lowest differentiation potential.

Mesenchymal vs Hematopoietic stem cells:

There is a very fine line between mesenchymal and hematopoietic stem cells. They are both found in the bone marrow and are multipotent. However, the mesenchymal cells are very few and give rise to other cells except blood cells, like osteoblasts (bone cells), adipose tissue (fat cells) and chondrocytes (cartilage cells). Hematopoietic stem cells differentiate into all the blood cell types. They are found in the 'red marrow', contained in the core of most bones.

Mesenchymal cells are also found in greater numbers in other tissues like adipose tissue, umbilical cord tissue, fallopian tube, fetal liver and lung. Morphologically, mesenchymal stem cells are long and possess thin cell bodies with a large nucleus. Like other stem cell types, MSCs have a high self-renewal capacity, are able to maintain multipotency. Therefore, mesenchymal stem cells have a vast therapeutic potential for tissue repair.

Hematopoietic stem cells are mainly found in the bone marrow (also called the red marrow) but are also found in the peripheral blood, umbilical cord blood and placenta. HSCs are the blood-forming cells. They proliferate and yield all types/lineages of blood cells comprising RBCs (red blood cells), WBCs (white blood cells), and platelets.

REFERENCES:

1. *Merriam-Webster's Learner's Dictionary*. (n.d.). Retrieved from Merriam-Webster Dictionary: http://www.merriam-webster.com/dictionary/stem%20cell

2. *Stem Cell Information*. (2016). Retrieved from NAtional Institutes of Health: https://stemcells.nih.gov/info/basics/1.htm

3. *About Stem cells*. (2005). Retrieved from Boston's Children Hospital: http://stemcell.childrenshospital.org/about-stem-cells/history/

4. *Childhood Diseases Treated with a Transplant*. (n.d.). Retrieved from **Seattle Cancer Care Alliance:** http://www.seattlecca.org/treatments/bone-mar-row-transplant/bone-marrow-transplant-facts/diseases-treated

5. K, H. (2011). Sources of human embryonic stem cells and ethics. *Medicina*, 1002-10

6. *Stem cell classification*. (n.d.). Retrieved from Biomed: http://biomed.brown.edu/Courses/BI108/BI108_2002_Groups/pancstems/stemcell/stem_cells-classes_2.htm

2

SOURCES OF STEM CELLS

FIND OUT WHERE THE STEM CELLS LIVE IN OUR BODY

Stem cells are called stem cells because they are where the rest of the cells of our body originate from. The cells that make up different tissues, muscles, organs, tracts and glands all 'stem' from stem cells. One of the fascinating facts about stem cells is that they serve as a 'back-up' for the back-up already provided by nature.

For instance, the human body replenishes its blood cell count through a 'negative feedback mechanism'. This is how the body tells itself something is wrong (the first back-up). Should a situation arise in which the cell count is decreased, warning signals are sent to the bone marrow indicating a shortage of cells in the circulation. This sets off the hematopoietic (blood-forming) stem cells into turbo mode (the second back-up). The rate of cell division and differentiation increases as does the turnover until the cell count in the circulation normalizes.

Having said this, thanks to advancements in Science and Technology and of course, tireless research, it is now a well-known fact that stem cells aren't only found in the bone marrow, but in other parts of the human body as well. Not only this, but they can be harvested or isolated from within the body only to be grown and/or modified in a laboratory for treatment of several critical illnesses like COPD and heart disease. This chapter will be dealing with the different sources of stem cells within the human body, how they are collected and what is done with them once they are in a science research lab.

The questions that surface most often in the field of stem cell therapy and research are:

- Where do scientists obtain the stem cells from?

- Where do stem cells reside in the human body?

This chapter will be dealing with these questions in as much detail as possible. As the saying goes, there is no such thing as a foolish question and answers only come to the questions that are asked. So here goes.

SCIENTISTS AND STEM CELLS

Almost half a century has passed since the first stem cell was discovered. Scientists have treasured their long-term relationship with the stem cell for the past so many years and continue to do so. After all, it has revolutionized medicinal therapy in unfathomable ways. Scientists continue to make leaps and bounds in stem cell research and technology and successful breakthrough therapies.

It is suggested that a stem cell is perhaps the most powerful cell of the human body. Its sophisticated nature never ceases to amaze scientists. Even after all these years of careful probing, there is still so much to learn and extract from them.

The profound value of a stem cell pertains to its regeneration and renewal potential among its many characteristics. The area of particular interest nowadays is how the exchange of signals and/or instructions causes a totipotent stem cell to differentiate into a pluripotent, multipotent, and unipotent cell, increasing its specialized function and restricting its potential at every step. By learning more about how these instructions work, in the future, scientists may be able to master this exchange of valuable information and manipulate the cells in a laboratory resulting in modification and growth of required stem cells.

While modified stem cells are being researched extensively, the increase of stem cell concentration in the body as well as their direct placement inside different tissues is the basis of current stem cell therapy.

SOURCES OF ADULT STEM CELLS

Adult stem cells are no longer under the radar. They have been a subject of interest for scientists, right alongside ESCs. Although they have a limited potential, their specialized function is what makes them useful in target-specific therapies. However, harvesting them is just the first step. They have to be infused in large numbers in order to be beneficial for therapy.

There are many sources of adult stem cells. The common ones are:

1. Bone marrow

2. Peripheral blood

3. Umbilical cord blood

4. Adipose tissue

Other sources include menstrual blood, skin, teeth, gut, liver, and brain. We will not discuss them in this book, since we consider them unavailable and impractical to use. It is also difficult to maintain sterility when collection is possible, and processing is complicated and expensive. Hence, currently they are not useful for stem cell therapy.

Adult stem cells found inside organs are 'tissue-specific stem cells that generate the type of tissue in which they are found'. [1] Adult stem cells found outside the vital organs can regenerate different kind of tissues of the same lineage, and because they are multipotent they can "jump" to other lineages, if surrounded by the proper stimulant factors.

1. BONE MARROW STEM CELLS:

The bone marrow is a dense fluid, inside a soft sponge like tissue. It is found in the hollow space of the bones' interior. It is perhaps the lightest tissue of the body, contributing only 4 % of the total body weight. There are two types of bone marrow, namely the red marrow and the yellow marrow.

While the function of red marrow is to produce the red blood cells, platelets, and majority of white blood cells; the yellow marrow serves as a fat reserve and among other functions produces cartilage and bone. The bone marrow is also a part of the lymphatic system.

There are two types of stem cells within the bone marrow:

i.   Hematopoietic stem cells, which are blood-forming stem cells.

ii.   Stromal stem cells, which form the stroma. The stroma is a fibrous tissue that supports the blood-forming stem cells.

All types of blood cells arise from one common stem cell. This common stem cell gives rise to two multipotent stem cells. One stem cell forms a lineage of red blood cells and platelets, while the other forms a lineage of most white cells. Therefore, the bone marrow basically consists of cells at various stages of development [8]

It is worth mentioning here that the bone marrow stroma consists of multipotent stem cells as well. They have the ability to differentiate into bone cells, cartilage cells, muscle cells, and fat cells. The stroma is not directly associated with blood cell formation. [8]

The stem cells are removed from the bone marrow by bone marrow aspiration. A needle is inserted into a big bone of the body, typically the back of the iliac bone (iliac crest), and then the bone marrow is aspirated. The patient is given a local/general anesthetic prior to the procedure. This procedure is invasive and carries with it the risk of infection. Nowadays, bone marrow aspiration is performed in the proper setup of a surgery room and with the expertise of doctors the risk of infection is minimal. When around a 100 ml of bone marrow or less is aspirated, patients may begin to feel uncomfortable. It becomes painful when high volumes of bone marrow is needed (like for a leukemia transplant), because several "drillings" are needed to get a certain number of "chambers" of bone in order to aspirate more than 300 ml.

The biggest advantage by far of using bone marrow stem

cells is that there is minimal risk of complications since the donor and recipient are the same (autologous transplantation). Autologous transplantation will be discussed in detail later in the book.

Other advantages include:

- High proliferation capacity

- High differentiation ability

- Low risk of viral contamination

- Autologous transplantation capacity

- No risk of tumor formation

Due to its differentiating potential, these stem cells are being used to treat immunological degenerative conditions, metabolic conditions, and others linked to the ageing process.

After extensive isolation preparation, bone marrow stem cells are introduced into the patient by the following methods:

i.   Intravenous

ii.   Intramuscular

iii. Intrajoint

iv.   Retrobulbar

v.   Intrathecal

vi.   Local deposition

2. PERIPHERAL BLOOD STEM CELLS:

The peripheral blood also contains hematopoietic stem cells similar to the bone marrow, but substantially in less quantity.

Stem cells that are removed from the peripheral blood require administration of injections of a particular drug that tells the bone marrow to 'spill' some of the stem cells into the circulation. The drug is a growth factor. It causes the bone marrow to increase production of stem cells. [9]

After the injection is given for a few days, a sufficient number of stem cells circulate in the bloodstream. The blood is then removed from a vein of an arm and passed through an apheresis machine. Each session on the machine takes 3-4 hours while it separates the stem cells from the blood. The blood is then passed back into the patient's body through a tube inserted in the other arm. This procedure is minimally invasive and carries minimal risk otherwise. There are a few secondary side effects of the drug and the apheresis process that could arise in some people and should be considered, such as muscle pain, hepatic toxicity and allergic reactions to anticoagulation factors. It is a widely used and popular method of donating or collecting blood-forming stem cells for bone marrow transplants.

Due to its differentiating potential, these stem cells are being used to treat immunological conditions, and some orthopedic conditions. In some cases, they are also useful to treat skin injuries such as diabetic foot.

After extensive isolation and preparation, bone marrow stem cells are introduced into the patient by the following methods:

i.   Intravenous

ii.   Intramuscular

iii. Intrajoint

iv.   Retrobulbar

v.   Intrathecal

vi.   Local deposition

3. UMBILICAL CORD BLOOD STEM CELLS:

The umbilical cord serves as a connection between the developing embryo and the placenta. It is also called the 'naval string' or the 'birth cord'.[3]

It consists of two umbilical arteries and one umbilical vein concealed within Wharton's jelly, a gelatinous substance that provides support to the blood vessels. The umbilical arteries carry the deoxygenated blood away from the fetus while the umbilical vein carries oxygenated blood to the fetus. It serves as a conduit for the exchange of oxygen and nutrients between the mother and fetus keeping both circulatory systems separated.

The umbilical cord forms around the 5th week of development and increases in length in proportion to fetal growth. At birth, the navel (umbilicus) marks the point of attachment of the umbilical cord during intrauterine life. In response to temperature and other changes in the baby's environment after birth, the umbilical cord constricts and closes naturally.

It can be mentioned here that during the viability phase of the fetus, i.e. 24-34 weeks, cord blood samples can be taken to test for hereditary abnormalities prior to birth. The doctor is likely to suggest it, if something 'isn't right'.

Umbilical cord blood is rich in blood-forming stem cells (blood cell precursors). Cord blood has proved extremely valuable in treating certain blood diseases like leukemia and lymphoma along with autoimmune diseases like aplastic anemia. The blood is transplanted into patients, so the precursor cells can form healthy cells and replace the blood cells that have been damaged by disease. Or in case of blood cancers, chemotherapy is used to eliminate cancer cells and wipe out the damaged bone marrow. The stem cells are then administered to the patient, replacing the bone marrow producing healthy new blood cells. The cord blood is collected quite easily into a collection bag, with no risk to the mother or baby.

Because of the risk involved in aspirating bone marrow from a child, the use of cord blood is a favorite for stem cell therapy in children. It also has the advantage of:

- High proliferation capacity

- High differentiation ability

- Autologous transplantation capacity

- No risk of tumor formation

Having said this, treating adults with cord blood poses a problem, only because they require a greater quantity of blood, which is not met by using blood from a single cord. That is why, double cord blood transplantation is used to treat adults for blood diseases. There is little evidence of cord blood cells being used for non-blood diseases.[5]

New research suggests that the umbilical cord tissue consists of mesenchymal stem cells.[10]

These stem cells are multipotent cells and are able to differentiate into a variety of cell types. Thus, allowing them to be used as a basis for regenerative therapy for a broad spectrum of conditions such as: [2]

- Skeletal disease

- Muscle injury

- Degenerative heart and vascular disease

- Neurological disease

- Diabetes

4. ADIPOSE TISSUE STEM CELLS:

Adipose tissue is also called fatty tissue. It is a type of connective tissue that comprises of fat cells or adipocytes. Connective tissue provides support and form to the body. Other examples of connective tissue include ligaments and tendons. Adipocytes are specialized cells, which produce large globules of fat.

Mostly, adipose tissues are present under the skin, but some are also deposited in the spaces between different muscles, around organs, and are associated with membrane folds of the intestines.

Since the basic function of fat is that of an energy store, so adipose tissue comes from two sources:

- Diet- Food we eat

- From within the body

Some of the dietary fat is broken down into carbohydrates and stored in the liver as a source of instant energy. The leftover fat is stored in the adipose tissue.

When the body endures a stressful state like starvation, the fat is consumed, by breaking it down and converting it into a form of usable energy.

Research now shows that adipose tissue stores a big amount of mesenchymal stem cells too. As mentioned earlier, they are multipotent in nature, i.e. they can differentiate into multiple cell lineages. This characteristic makes them favorites for regenerative medicinal therapy. Other favorable characteristics include:

• Present in abundant quantity

• Minimally invasive harvesting

• Are safe to use in autologous and allogeneic host

• Can be manufactured according to GMP guidelines (good manufacturing practices)

• The use in allogeneic cases, have shown little to no immunologic reaction.

Adipose stem cells are extracted via liposuction or needle aspiration. Although it is minimally invasive, there are still risks involved in the collection, and side effects post procedure.

Like bone marrow stem cells, they too can differentiate into chondrocytes (cartilage), osteocytes (bone cells), neurogenic (brain cells), myocytes (muscle cells) and of course adipocytes.[6]

Due to its differentiating potential, these stem cells are being used to treat osteoarthritis and other musculoskeletal conditions linked to the ageing process.

After extensive isolation preparation, adipose stem cells are introduced into the patient by the following methods:

i.   Intravenous

ii. Intramuscular

iii. Intrajoint

iv. Local deposition

Adipose stem cell research is being prodded now more than ever as an effective means of treating patients through autologous and allogeneic transplants as compared to other sources of stem cells.

SOURCES OF EMBRYONIC STEM CELLS

Currently, embryonic stem cells are not being used in stem cell therapy. They are controversial because of the ethical issues involved in their collection, religious matters, and in many countries they are illegal. Also, there are several unwanted risks involved, such as forming solid tumors or interfering with the immunologic system. We mention them below as a reference because they are a source of stem cells.

1. USING EXISTING EMBRYOS TO HARVEST EMBRYONIC STEM CELLS:

This process has always had its share of controversy over the years. Having said this, it is the most widely accepted method of obtaining ESCs.[4]

The argument that stands is that using a stem cell line that already exists in its natural form is the best approach to obtain accurate results.

2. USING LEFT-OVER EMBRYOS FROM FERTILITY TREATMENTS

This technique too is much disputed over by different schools of thought. During fertility treatments, it is common for unused, spare embryos being 'left behind'. The argument here is that if they aren't going to be transplanted in a womb, they can't grow into a human in a petri dish. So, with relative consent, the proper thing to do would be to use it for research purposes.

3. USING SOMATIC CELL NUCLEAR TRANSFER (SCNT):

The very famous Dolly sheep was produced using this seemingly complicated technique. It's actually quite simple. A somatic cell is any cell of the body besides the sperm or the egg. The nucleus of a somatic cell is removed as is the nucleus of an egg/ovum. The nucleus contains the organism's DNA (in this case a sheep). The egg acts as a host cell. A host cell is defined as a 'living cell invaded by or capable of being invaded by another agent.' [7]

The somatic cell nucleus is transferred into the enucleated egg resulting in the reprogramming of the somatic cell nucleus by the host cell. The egg will now start to divide and after a series of divisions will produce a blastocyst-like it would under normal circumstances. The blastocyst cells consist of DNA, which is identical to the organism the nucleus was harvested from.

As mentioned in the previous chapter, a blastocyst is the primary source of ESCs.

REFERENCES

1.   Adult Stem Cell 101. (2015-2016). *WHERE DO WE GET ADULT STEM CELLS?* Retrieved from Boston Children's Hospital: http://stemcell.children-shospital.org/about-stem-cells/adult-somatic-stem-cells-101/where-do-we-get-adult-stem-cells/

2.   Cord Blood Registry. (1995-2016). *What is Cord Tissue?* Retrieved from cbr: http://www.cordblood.com/benefits-cord-blood/cord-tissue

3.   Douglas Harper. (2016). *Online Etymology Dictionary.* Retrieved from Online Etymology Dictionary: http://www.etymonline.com/index

4.   hp?frame=0&search=Umbilical+&searchmode=none

5.   EuroStemCell . (2015, November 5). *Origins, ethics and embryos: the sources of human embryonic stem cells.* Retrieved from EuroStemCell: http://www.eurostemcell.org/factsheet/origins-ethics-and-embryos-sources-human-embryonic-stem-cells

6.   Gupta, R. (2016, March 03). *Cord blood stem cells: current uses and future challenges.* Retrieved from EuroStemCell: http://www.eurostemcell.org/factsheet/cord-blood-stem-cells-current-uses-and-future-challenges

7.   Lindroos B, S. R. (2011). The potential of adipose stem cells in regenerative medicine. *PubMEd* , 269-91.

8.   Merriam-Webster. (n.d.). *Meidcal Dictionary.* Retrieved from Merriam-Webster Dictionary: www.merriam-webster.com

9.   Panchbhavi, V. K. (2015, July 21). *Bone Marrow Anatomy.* Retrieved from Medscape: http://emedicine.medscape.com/article/1968326-overview#a3

10.   PubMed Health. (2013, november 11). *How are blood stem cells obtained for transplantation?* Retrieved from PubMed Health: http://www.ncbi.nlm.nih.gov/pubmedhealth/PMH0072612/

11.   Trounson A, T. R. (2011). Clinical Trials for Stem Cell Therapies. *BMC Medicine.*

3

WHY STEM CELLS ARE PREFERRED FOR THERAPY

A question that arises in the minds of many would be 'why are stem cells favored for replacement or regeneration therapy?' Why not other types of cells? If the body has so many cells to choose from then what makes stem cells so special?

Well, there is a wide array of properties that stem cells possess which renders them unique as compared to other cells. Some significant traits will be discussed in this chapter, which will provide a better understanding of why stem cells are the most suitable for cell replacement therapy.

The most basic definition of a stem cell would be a cell from which all other cells arise. However, oversimplification often results in confusion and leads to more questions than answers. In terms of functionality, a stem cell is one which has a self-renewal ability, i.e. it can form progenitor cells that are identical to the mother cell, as well as differentiating ability by which it can give rise to different types of cell lineages.

Among these two traits, is the potency and replication capacity. [1] As mentioned earlier, potency is the potential of a stem cell to produce differentiated progeny. The more differentiated the cells are, the more they are specialized in terms of function.

Replication capacity is a cell's inherent ability to duplicate. For instance, research suggests that a somatic cell (in vitro) replicates into about 80 cells before ceasing to divide, whereas a stem cell has an ability to divide into an infinite number of cells. In other words, these cells are proficient and extensive proliferators, a trait also known as self-renewal.

This chapter is going to highlight four significant characteristics of stem cells:

1. Stemness

2. Homing

3. Self-renewal

4. Differentiation

Stemness:

Stemness is a quality which is unique to all stem cells. It is a trait that sets apart stem cells from other cells. It is known that stem cells are inherently unspecialized cells and stemness refer to their ability to generate more unspecialized cells by self-renewal yet retaining the ability to produce specialized cells as well.

The somatic (specialized) cells of the human body eventually wear, tear, or die out and need to be replaced by new cells. Stem cell proliferation provides an appropriate supply of differentiated cells for the sustenance of specialized tissue.

For instance, the average life span of a normal red blood cell is about 120 days. Once a red cell dies, the blood-forming stem cells in the bone marrow not only form more stem cells, but red blood cell progenitors as well, which eventually develop into mature red cells in the circulation. The same principle is followed by stem cells in different tissues of the body. The function will depend on the stem cell niche. [2]

Despite stemness being an apparently common characteristic of all stem cells, it is much more complex at the molecular level. At present, stem cells largely differentiate into the corresponding cell niche in which they reside. This means that a stem cell from one niche may have some difficulty in being exchanged with a stem cell from another niche for regenerative purposes. This may prove to be a limitation in advanced cellular therapy.

Researchers and scientists are trying to find a common gene among stem cells, regardless of their niche, so they may be used universally. It is postulated that there is probably a 'stemness gene' which is mutual among all stem cells. However, scientists face certain technical difficulties in experiments and aren't quite there yet. [3] But nonetheless, stem cells are still used effectively in a wide array of regenerative therapies.

Stem cells are usually harvested from younger tissues. This can be explained better by comparing the process with a tree. The goal is to obtain stem cells at the "trunk" stage. The immature cells further specialize into a "branch" and sub-specialize into "twigs" to finally become a functional cell of a specific tissue, or a "leaf".

Homing:

Homing is a complex but controlled process by which stem cells navigate their way through the body to reach their tissue of origin. It is perhaps the most important step in the process of stem cell transplantation. The precision of the homing process is controlled by multiple chemokines (chemical stimuli) produced by the cells in the microenvironment. They 'guide' the stem cells at various stages of navigation until they reach the desired destination. For instance, very late antigen 4/5 (VLA-4/5), lymphocyte function–associated antigen 1 (LFA-1) and stem cell factor (SCF) are just a few examples of regulatory cytokines.

HOMING OF HEMATOPOIETIC STEM CELLS.

Complete Stem cell transplantation is most widely used in various forms of blood cancer such as leukemia. Effective stem cell transplantation comprises of three main stages:

- Homing

- Engraftment

- Repopulation

Hematopoietic stem cells are usually introduced by the intravascular route. It is essential to determine the range of chemokines prior to stem cell administration that will aid in organ-specific stem cell homing.

Once the stem cells are in circulation, certain chemokines help the stem cells find their way 'home', which in this case is the bone marrow.

HOMING IS MADE UP OF A SEQUENCE OF EVENTS:

i. Rolling

ii. Adhesion

iii. Transmigration

Rolling:

The initial stage is called **rolling**, which is the linking of a stem cell to a vascular endothelial cell (the epithelial cells that line the blood vessel) mediated by a chemokine known as E-selectin. The rolling process invites a cluster of stem cells at the vascular endothelium by slowing some of the cells down and separating them from the faster ones in circulation. [4]

Adhesion:

Once a stem cell has formed a connection with a vascular endothelial cell, adhesion takes place. Adhesion as the name suggests, is the physical union of a stem cell with an endothelial cell. This step prepares a stem cell for the next and final step of homing i.e. transmigration.

Transmigration:

Transmigration is the process by which a stem cell crosses the endothelial membrane and enters the organs/bone marrow. Research suggests that this progression across the membrane is mediated by a certain transmembrane adhesion molecule known as CD44.

As a result, homing of the bone marrow is essential for optimal cell engraftment. [5]

Self-Renewal

In order to classify a cell as a true stem cell, it must possess the ability to perform several cycles of cell division while still retaining the undifferentiated state. This process is known as self-renewal and is by far the most significant property of a stem cell which preserves a constant pool of stem cells throughout life. This characteristic renders stem cells as the most favorable for cell regeneration therapy as they not only have the ability to produce more stem cells but also differentiate into specialized cells when need be.

Cell division is a controlled phenomenon and is kept in check by various chemical regulators. This is important in terms of preventing overgrowth and excess of cells. The self-renewal system is balanced by the following three major components:

- Proto-oncogenes that stimulate self-renewal

- Gatekeeping tumor suppressors that limit self-renewal

- Care-taking tumor suppressors that maintain genomic integrity [6]

At the microscopic level, the changes that go on within the cell are actually controlled by regulators present outside the cell in the microenvironment that sustains stem cells and regulates their function in tissues. The habitat of a stem cell is known as a stem cell niche.

Stem cells renew and duplicate variably, depending on

tissue demand. The stem cell division cycle and developmental potential alter over time calling for diverse self-renewal programs at different stages of life.

As age progresses, the self-renewal process, as well as the tissue regeneration capacity, slow down. Certain changes cause an escalation in tumor suppression. Wild or incongruous self-renewal activation, however, could result in tumors. [6]

Differentiation

Differentiation, as described in the previous chapters, is the ability of a stem cell to produce a specialized cell by multiple cell divisions. This network is regulated by specific chemokines that direct a stem cell at every stage. As the level of differentiation progresses the cell potential is decreased. Cell function, however, is directly proportional to the level of differentiation. Highly differentiated cells are more specialized. This unique characteristic of stem cells makes it extremely efficient for target based regenerative therapy. A stem cell can be manipulated in vitro, resulting in the controlled growth and development or by placing the stem cell in the microenvironment (surrounding cells) where regeneration is needed.

Clinical Application:

TISSUE REPAIR:

A specific type of tissue could be 'grown' in a laboratory and be used as a tissue source for transplantation therapy to repair damaged or dead tissue.

RESEARCH:

Scientists and researchers use stem cells to grow a specific cell type for research purposes. For instance, scientists have used stem cells from Parkinson's patients to grow neurons so they can study why neurons die in Parkinson's disease.

COMPLETE TRANSPLANTATION THERAPY:

Highly differentiated specialized stem cells are used to treat a variety of diseases. For instance, blood cancers such as leukemia are treated by eliminating the cancer cells with chemotherapy and radiation. It is so aggressive that the immune system of the patient is compromised. Therefore, a complete bone marrow transplant or stem cell transplant is performed, which consists of hematopoietic or blood-forming stem cells. Hematopoietic stem cells then differentiate into different lineages resulting in the formation of the cellular components of the blood, i.e. red blood cells, white blood cells, and platelets, rescuing the patient by creating a new immune system.

DEGENERATIVE DISEASES:

Also known as partial stem cell transplant, bone marrow/ adipose tissue are extracted and then processed in an advanced laboratory to isolate stem cells and yield specific cell types for therapy. For example, heart disease can be treated by using undifferentiated stem cells that differentiate into the cardiac tissue increasing efficiency in the organ.

These are just a few applications of stem cells and their therapeutic use in the scientific realm. New properties are constantly being discovered and new processes unleashed. Stem cell therapy is revolutionizing the way patients with complex diseases are being treated.

The above-mentioned hallmark characteristics are not seen in any other cell type. It is an eye-opening discovery and there is much more to unveil. Having said this, the information out there at the moment is saving lives already and the future holds great prospects.

REFERENCES:

1.   Melton, D. (n.d.). 'Stemness': Definitions, Criteria. In D. Melton. Harvard
     University, Cambridge, MA, USA: Department of Molecular and Cellular
     Biology and Howard Hughes Medical Institute.

2.   Pedersen, P. R. (2007, October 28). Stem Cells and 'Stemness'. (Chris, Inter-
     viewer)

3.   Cai, J., Weiss, M. and Rao, M. (2004). In search of "stemness". *Experimental
     Hematology*, 32(7), pp.585-598.

4.   Khaldoyanidi, S. (2008). Direct Stem Cell Homing. *Cell Stem Cell*, 2(3),
     pp.198-200.

5.   Suárez-Álvarez, B., López-Vázquez, A. and López-Larrea, C. (2012). Mo-
     bilization and Homing of Hematopoietic Stem Cells. *Advances in Experimental
     Medicine and Biology*, pp.152-170. Doi: 10.1007/978-1-4614-2098-9_11

6.   Shenghui, H., Nakada, D. and Morrison, S. (2009). Mechanisms of Stem
     Cell Self-Renewal. *Annual Review of Cell and Developmental Biology*, 25(1),
     pp.377-406. doi: 10.1146/annurev.cellbio.042308.113248.

4

THE PROCESS OF STEM CELL THERAPY

HOW TO HARVEST STEM CELLS AND ADMINISTER THEM

Stem cell therapy has not only been a groundbreaking discovery in the realm of regenerative therapy, but it is proving to be an inventive space for researchers, doctors, and scientists. Since everything is manipulated and monitored at a cellular level, researchers often cross paths with certain challenges when it comes to precision and efficacy. At the same time, they have to make sure that the benefits of stem cell therapy outweigh the risks.

Everything from the harvesting of stem cells to the administration and the follow-ups requires great skill and accuracy. This chapter will be highlighting the different methods by which stem cells are collected, the various sites at which they reside, and different modes of their administration to the patient.

It is the ethical responsibility of the doctor to counsel the patient about the procedure before beginning the process. Most likely any decent doctor or clinic will provide a patient with a document called informed consent, reviewed by an ethical committee (IRB). This informed consent explains exactly all medical procedures that the patient will go through, as well tests, exams, secondary effects, risks, alternative treatments, and many other important information. This also gives the patient an opportunity to raise any questions or concerns, if needed. Research suggests that patients with a positive attitude have a better overall prognosis.

The main sources of stem cell collection are:

1. Bone marrow

2. Adipose tissue

3. Cord blood in newborns

4. Peripheral blood

BONE MARROW STEM CELL HARVEST

OVERVIEW OF BONE MARROW

As mentioned in the previous chapters, the bone marrow is a spongy and fatty tissue found in the core of bones. The bone marrow has one of the most important functions in the human body in terms of sustaining the physiology of the circulatory system, i.e. it is responsible for the production of blood cells.

The bone marrow consists of blood-forming stem cells that divide and differentiate into three main lineages:

- Red blood cells, which transport oxygen to the whole body

- White blood cells, which are part of the immune system and help fight off infections

- Platelets, which help in blood clotting [1]

INDICATIONS OF BONE MARROW ASPIRATION

One of the most important applications of bone marrow aspiration is to harvest stem cells for a stem cell therapy. It is used by doctors and researchers to determine whether the treatment is effective and/or to evaluate the side effects of chemotherapy. In the past 15 years, bone marrow stem cells have shown not only differentiation into blood forming cells but also have been determined to help into creating some chemical signals to help the body create other kind of cells such as cartilage, internal organs tissue, and even neurons when situated next of the brain barrier; in addition they help to regulate the immune system and trigger the regeneration process of damaged cells.

Bone marrow aspiration could be useful for the diagnosis of a variety of diseases such as:

- Blood diseases, like leukemia, lymphoma, multiple myelomas etc.

- Fever of unknown origin

- Stem cell disorders

- Metastatic and primary tumors

- Cause of anemia

SITES OF BONE MARROW ASPIRATION

A bone marrow sample is usually collected from the back of the pelvic bone (posterior iliac crest). This site is preferred, as it does not harbor any major blood vessels, nerves, or organs. An alternative site of the pelvic bone anterior iliac crest is the tibia bone (inferior leg bone), it is very near the skin without major vessels or nerves to be in the way to access the spongy bone.

Sometimes, the bone on the anterior chest wall, the sternum, is used, although it is a superficial structure, but it is painful and poses a greater risk due to the close proximity of the heart and major blood vessels.

PROCEDURE

A small bone marrow aspiration from the hipbone could be very simple and painless when performed by an expert. In an operating room under sterile conditions, the donor is given a local anesthetic and the harvesting of stem cells takes place. The time varies from person to person, however, the procedure takes about 20 min. An aspiration needle is inserted once into the marrow cavity of one the hipbones and a big syringe aspirate the inside of the bone getting bone marrow. The discomfort or pain reported by patients are in the range of 4 to 5 in a 0 to 10 level (being 10 very painful). It is very tolerable, patients mention the discomfort lasts less than 20 seconds.

The donor is likely to experience little discomfort when the anesthesia fades off at the entry site, and will remain for a couple of days after the procedure. Usually the discomfort is very tolerable so no analgesics are needed except for very sensitive patients.

People often get confused with a complete stem cell transplant where a painful bone marrow aspiration from the hip bone is done. Also the harvesting of stem cells takes place in an operating room under sterile conditions but this time the donor is given a general anesthetic (patient must consider the risks and side effects of general anesthesia). The procedure time of aspiration varies but takes at least an hour. An ideal position for bone marrow aspiration is the prone position. An aspiration needle is inserted into the marrow cavity of the hip bone. It takes multiple punctures on both hip bones to collect an adequate amount of bone marrow. [2]

The donor is likely to experience pain at both hips for several days after the procedure. The pain is often relieved by over the counter analgesics.

ADVANTAGES

- Minimum negative side effects

- Painless when done by an experienced doctor

- No ethical issues

- Sterile

- Fast post-operative recovery

- Fewer complications

- General anesthesia is not required

- Outpatient procedure

DISADVANTAGES

- Not recommended for small bones such as with infants

- Not recommended when patients have anemia, or blood clotting problems (people with blood thinners have could have complications).

ADIPOSE TISSUE STEM CELL HARVEST

OVERVIEW OF ADIPOSE TISSUE

Adipose tissue is a type of loose connective tissue which consists of adipocytes or fat cells, thus, also known as fatty tissue. Its main function is to store energy in the form of fat. It is also known as the insulator of the body. The adipose tissue found under the skin keeps the body warm. It also surrounds vital organs, protecting them from surrounding structures.

Adipose-derived stem cells. The stem cells, which reside in adipose tissue differ from embryonic stem cells in terms of differentiation potential. Adipose-derived stem cells are mesenchymal stem cells. They are pluripotent in nature, i.e. they are able to differentiate into cells of ectodermal, endodermal, and mesodermal origin. They have the ability to develop into multiple cell lineages regardless of the tissue of origin. Hence, mesenchymal stem cells possess functional properties of cells unique to other tissues. Such stem cells can be extracted from various tissues, such as the brain, gut, liver, bone marrow, and adipose tissue. [5]

Adipose tissue is derived from the embryonic mesenchyme, hence, contains a stroma consisting of mesenchymal stem cells, which can be accessed easily. Therefore, the adipose tissue serves as a great source of stem cells with great potential for a variety of regenerative therapies. [6]

PROCEDURE

MINI LIPOSUCTION:

The most common site of stem cell harvest from adipose tissue is the abdominal wall. A local anesthetic is administered to the abdominal area and a mini liposuction is performed. The procedure is performed by trained and skilled personnel. An aspiration needle is used to extract the fat. The amount of fat removed will depend on the procedure, it is needed for, but usually 40-200cc of fat is removed. Adipose tissue is aspirated from both sides of the abdomen to ensure a symmetrical distribution of fat. It is a half an hour procedure on average. It is very important to mention that this type of mini liposuction is not an esthetical procedure like a plastic surgeon will perform to contour the body. In those cases much more fat volume is removed therefore other medical implications are in place, such as higher risk and longer recovery.

SEPARATION:

The samples are collected in test tubes and sent to the lab for further processing. In the lab, a test tube is placed in a centrifuge apparatus and spun at a varying speed and length of time to separate the stem cells. The end result is a test tube with fat concentrate on top and stem cells at the bottom of the test tube. The separation process also takes about another 30 minutes. The stem cells are then carefully removed from the test tube and are ready to be 'expanded' or 'enriched'.

EXPANSION AND/OR ENRICHMENT.

After having the isolated stem cells, there are a few techniques that could follow.   Some doctors will place them with platelet-rich blood derived from the donor. Platelets consist of one growth factor, which will help to activate the stem cells. Other doctors prefer to place them immersed in media and growth factors inside a CO_2 incubator to grow more cells, this is also called cultured cells, expanded cells or multiplicated cells, and the key is to avoid differentiation to preserve the potential of the cell.

Expanded cells can also be cryopreserved in special tanks with very low temperatures as low as -190°Celsius using liquid nitrogen. Cryopreserved cells can be stored for decades and be thawed for future procedures.

TREATMENT:

Now that the stem cells are fresh cultured, or enriched or thawed, they are washed to remove any reagent used in the process and are ready to be used for the treatment.

ADVANTAGES:

• Less ethical issues

- Adequate sample size can be obtained

- Adipose tissue that is discarded in elective surgeries can be useful

- Immune rejection is minimal, especially in an autologous transplant

- Outpatient procedure

- Minimal side effects

DISADVANTAGES:

- Painless during the procedure, but some analgesics are used when the anesthesia fades off

- Antibiotic is recommended to prevent any infection.

- Abdominal recovery can take up to 20 days to eliminate liquids and healing the tissue under the skin. Purple and red areas of the skin will turn back to original color after this time.

- Remote risk of organ puncture

CORD BLOOD STEM CELL HARVEST

OVERVIEW OF THE UMBILICAL CORD AND CORD BLOOD

The umbilical cord or birth cord is the structure that connects the fetus with the womb of the mother during pregnancy. It serves as a conduit for the exchange and transport of oxygen and nutrients between maternal and fetal circulations. After birth, the cord is clamped, cut, and discarded along with the placenta. However, not too long ago, it was discovered that cord blood was a rich source of stem cells.

Cord blood stem cells are being used to treat blood and immune diseases. They help regenerate healthy blood and strengthen the immune system. Research suggests that cord blood stem cells have been used in over 35000 transplants worldwide. [7]

PROCEDURE.

After the birth of a baby, the cord blood is left within the umbilical cord and placenta. It is collected via a syringe/needle, causing no harm to the mother or baby. The sample is then stored or frozen for future use, a term known as 'cord blood banking'.

ADVANTAGES

- Easily accessible

- Causes no harm to mother or baby

- Not invasive

- No anesthesia is required

- Cord tissue can also be used to harvest stem cells

DISADVANTAGES

- Sample size is not that big (specially on multiple child pregnancies)

- Cord blood banking could get expensive

- Only 1 opportunity to collect (during childbirth)

PERIPHERAL BLOOD STEM CELL HARVEST

Overview of peripheral blood

Peripheral blood refers to that in circulation. It consists of cells and plasma. The cellular component is made up of red blood cells, white blood cells, and platelets. The plasma is the liquid part of the blood which contains water, proteins, minerals and dissolved gases. The peripheral blood is normally devoid of stem cells, however, stem cells can be mobilized from bone marrow into circulation by administration of certain drugs.

PROCEDURE

A couple of days prior to collection, the donor usually receives injections of a mobilizing drug which transfers the stem cells into the peripheral blood circulation from the bone marrow. Most people tolerate the drugs quite well, however, flu-like symptoms may be experienced. A daily dose ensures that a sufficient amount of stem cells has mobilized into the circulating blood.

MECHANISM OF ACTION

The drugs force the bone marrow to 'purge' stem cells into the circulation by two methods:

- Large doses of chemotherapy are given to the donor which kills off most of the white blood cells. This deficit of white blood cells in the circulation signals the bone marrow to go into 'overdrive' to replenish them. Like this, the abundance of white blood cell progenitors is forced into the blood stream.

- A growth factor like G-CSF (granulocyte-colony stimulating factor) can also be administered. This causes rapid maturation of stem cells into neutrophils (a particular type of white blood cell). Since there is not enough space in the marrow cavity for the excess neutrophils, stem cells are forced into the circulation to make a room for the new cells. [3]

On the day of harvest, the donor is seated comfortably on a chair and two IV lines are maintained on each arm. The IV lines are connected to an apheresis machine. This is a special machine, which separates the stem cells from the cellular components of the blood. The blood is drawn from one arm and after separation, the blood is returned via the other arm. A central venous catheter may be used in case the veins are incapable of penetration. Each round of collection usually takes an average of 3 to 4 hours. However, this procedure is repeated for at least three days for collection of an adequate sample size. [4]

ADVANTAGES

- Speedy recovery

- Fewer major complications

- General anesthesia is not required

- The procedure can be repeated in case of inadequate sample size

- Outpatient procedure

DISADVANTAGES:

- Donor may experience mild to severe bone pain

- Donor may experience side effects such as dizziness, body pain, fatigue from the drugs that mobilizes the cells.

- Long procedure, not recommended for hyperactive people.

ROUTES OF STEM CELL ADMINISTRATION

Once stem cells are harvested, expanded and enriched, an appropriate route of administration has to be attained. This really depends on the procedure it is being used for.

The common routes of stem cell administration are:

INTRAVENOUS

This route is used for most stem cell transplants, particularly in blood cancers and immune diseases. This is the most common route because it will take stem cells all over the body where blood is found. It will be able to reach all organs, will create better blood circulation even creating new vessels and will have a great impact on the immunologic system. Patient is laying down or sitting and an I.V. through the arm delivers a solution rich in stem cells.

INTRATHECAL

This route is used in regenerative therapies of the spinal cord and neurological conditions. Research suggests that among physical and rehabilitative therapy, stem cell therapy has also shown to be effective in treating spinal cord injury. [9]   Cells are expected to be released on the spinal fluid, which in turn will take the stem cells all the way up to the brain, and wash the brain with them. There is still a lot of discussion if the stem cells could go through the brain barrier or if they stimulate from the outside of the barrier to create neuronal connections improving neurological conditions.   Stem cells are concentrated in a very small volume, and set into a syringe. A well-experienced doctor inserts the needle between 2 vertebras in the lumbar area and release the cells into the spinal fluid canal.

INTRA-JOINT

This route is used to treat degenerative conditions such as osteoarthritis, chondromalacia, osteoporosis, etc.   The most common places are the ones where cartilage needs to be regenerated such as direct injection to the knees, ankles and shoulders. Stem cells are concentrated in a small volume, and set into a syringe. A well-experienced doctor inserts the needle inside the joint bone structure and releases the cells.

RETROBULBAR.

This route, as the name suggests, is used to treat conditions of the eye like degenerative retinal, retinitis pigmentosa and macular degeneration. Stem cells are concentrated in a very small volume, and set into a syringe. A well experienced ophthalmologist inserts the needle below the eye ball releasing the stem cells in the back of the eye, near the optic nerve.

REFERENCES

1. *Bone Marrow Aspiration and Biopsy.* (2015). Retrieved from Cancer.Net: http://www.cancer.net/navigating-cancer-care/diagnosing-cancer/tests-and-procedures/bone-marrow-aspiration-and-biopsy

2. *Fat Stem Cell Therapy.* (2015). Retrieved from Infinite Horizons Medical Center: http://www.fatstemcelltherapy.com/procedure/

3. Munoz J, S. N. (2014). umbilical cord blood transplantation: past, present, and future. *Stem Cells Transl Med* , 1435-1443.

4. Patricia A. Zuk, *. M. (2002). Human Adipose Tissue Is a Source of Multipotent Stem Cells. *Molecular Biology of the Cell* , 4279–4295.

5. *Stem cell harvest procedure.* (2016). Retrieved from Non Hodgkin Lymphoma Cyberfamily: http://www.nhlcyberfamily.org/treatments/collection.htm#-methods

6. *Stem Cell Therapy and spinal cord injury.* (2016). Retrieved from Stem cell institute: https://www.cellmedicine.com/stem-cell-therapy-for-spinal-cord-injury/

7. *Stem Cell/Bone Marrow Collection.* (n.d.). Retrieved from Blood and Marrow transplant information network: http://www.bmtinfonet.org/before/stemcellmarrowharvest

8. Terskikh AV, E. M. (2001). From hematopoiesis to neuropoiesis: evidence of overlapping genetic programs. *Proc Natl Acad Sci U S A* , 7934-9.

9. *The Bone Marrow Harvest Procedure.* (1995-2016). Retrieved from Cleveland Clinic: http://my.clevelandclinic.org/health/treatments_and_procedures/hic_Bone_Marrow_and_Transplantation/hic-bone-marrow-harvest-procedure

5

ALTERNATIVE TREATMENT REGIMENS

ALTERNATIVE TREATMENT REGIMES TO AUGMENT THE STEM-CELL THERAPY

Stem cell therapy is a complex, multi-step procedure involving several biochemical and physiological alterations at a molecular level. It is a process that not only exerts stress on the cellular components of the human body, but in fact, compels it to adapt the ongoing changes in the micro-environment.

The different systems of the body are somewhat jolted at every step along the way. For instance, the administration of stem cell mobilizing drugs prior to stem cell harvest results the bone marrow to go into overdrive. The extra effort that the bone marrow exerts, may cause some discomfort and bone pain. Similarly, there are apparent and unapparent deviations, and fluctuations that the patient's body goes through at one level or another.

This chapter will go through certain alternative treatment regimens which will augment the process of stem cell therapy as they help in the maintenance of a healthy mind and body. If the cells and tissues are kept in optimal and healthy conditions before stem cell therapy is provided, it has been shown to reduce the discomfort, pain, and anxiety that a patient may experience.

The following are some of the tried and tested treatment therapies:

1. Ozone therapy

2. Hyperbaric Therapy

3. Nutritional plan

4. Physical activity

5. Detoxification Therapy or Chelation Therapy

OZONE THERAPY

As the name indicates, this therapy uses ozone for curative purposes. This may sounds impractical and dangerous, but the scientific explanation behind it relieves all the doubts.

Ozone therapy is the use of medicinal ozone or medically approved ozone, to create a therapeutic response in the body.

What is ozone?

Ozone is a highly reactive and unstable form of a pure oxygen. An ozone molecule consists of three atoms of oxygen (O_3). Medical ozone has been studied for more than a hundred years now, and the initial perception of it causes more harm than good has been disproved. In fact, research suggests that it has several therapeutic effects. [1]

What it is used for?

Ozone therapy is not only safe, but effective as-well, and with a few and preventable side effects. A wide spectrum of diseases is treated with ozone therapy, such as:

- Bacterial Infections

- Viral Infections

- Fungal Infections

- Protozoal Infections

- Cancer

- Infected wounds

- Circulatory conditions

- Macular degeneration

- Geriatric conditions

- Rheumatism/ Arthritis

- SARS

- AIDS

Mechanism of Action:

Inactivation. Ozone therapy halts the disease process by inactivating the relative microorganisms, i.e. bacteria, viruses, fungi, protozoa, etc. For instance, in bacterial infections, ozone molecules destroy the bacterial cell wall, and similarly, the viral capsid in viral infections. In fungal infections, fungal growth is inhibited. The weakened cells are then susceptible to oxidation and elimination, after which they are replaced by the healthy cells.

Acceleration of Oxygen Metabolism. Ozone therapy stimulates several biochemical changes, and incites increased oxygen release to the tissues as well as an increase in ATP production. ATP is the basic unit of energy required for cell function.

Boost of immune system. When ozone is administered in a specific range (30-50 micrograms/cc), it causes an increased release of TNF (tumor necrosis factor), IL-2 (Interleukin-2), and interferon. This further results in a surge of immunological responses. [1]

How is ozone used to treat cancer?

Ozone therapy works well for certain cancers as it is a highly targeted option, leaving very little margin for inefficiency. Cancer cells are anaerobic in nature, i.e., they don't require oxygen for survival. Since ozone consists of highly active oxygen particles, the cancer cells begin to die when exposed to oxygen.

There are two widely used techniques for ozone therapy:

- Bottle Infusion Therapy: In this method, an infusion bottle is filled with the patient's blood, after which ozone is administered to the bottle. The treated blood within the infusion bottle is infused back into the patient. The oxygen molecules target the cancer cells within the body.

- I.V. Infusion Therapy: This method works on the same

principle, except that there is no extraction of blood. An ozone saturated concoction is given to the patient intravenously. [2]

HYPERBARIC THERAPY

WHAT IS HYPERBARIC OXYGEN?

Hyperbaric medicine refers to the use of oxygen at levels higher than atmospheric pressure (three times the normal atmospheric pressure), hence, also known as hyperbaric oxygen therapy (HBOT). Under normal circumstances, when oxygen is administered to a patient, Hb (hemoglobin) in the blood takes it up and distributes it to all the body tissues. However, when 100% oxygen is used, the Hb becomes saturated and when it is unable to take up any more oxygen. The free oxygen then accumulates in the plasma. This phenomenon is known as hyper-oxygenation of the blood.

WHAT IS IT USED FOR?

Hyperbaric oxygen therapy is used for a plethora of conditions, and because it acts on the root of the problem, it is shown to have astounding results. Normal tissues require an adequate amount of oxygen to keep them healthy. When a tissue is injured, it is hungry for even more oxygen in order to survive. Hyperbaric oxygen fulfills this need. [7]

The following are some of the conditions for which hyperbaric therapy is used successfully:

• Wound injury

- Severe anemia

- Abscess

- Sudden deafness

- Sudden loss of vision

- Gangrene

- Burns

- Decompression sickness

- Carbon monoxide poisoning

- Crushing injury

- Arterial gas embolism

How is hyperbaric oxygen therapy used?

Hyperbaric oxygen therapy is usually an outpatient procedure. Most therapy sessions last for about two hours. The time duration may vary depending on the condition. It is administered via two basic types of chambers:

- Monoplace Chamber: As the name indicates, a monoplace chamber treats one person at a time. The patient is usually compressed with 100% oxygen. Sometimes, there may be an alternative outlet for breathable oxygen within the chamber (such as air). The rest of the equipment and attendees remain outside the compression chamber.

- Multiplace Chamber: This chamber is designed to

treat many people at the same time. The patients in a multiplace chamber breathe in the hyperbaric oxygen through a tube or a hood that covers the head. A nurse/attendant accompanies the patients inside the room and monitors them. [3]

NUTRITIONAL PLAN

This is not an unknown secret or some recent revelation that diet plays an immensely important role in not only keeping the body fit, but also protects the body from harmful agents, and prepares it for unprecedented weakness. The importance of a good diet before and after stem cell transplantation cannot be undermined in any way.

Stem cell transplants take a toll on one's body even before they are administered. Cancer is one of the most common conditions for which a stem cell therapy is used. Cancer, more often than not, renders a patient weak and malnourished. Physicians take care of the overall health of the patient in an attempt to attend the more serious problems at hand. However, research suggests that this is a huge loophole. The overall well-being of the patient has been just as important as the acute signs and symptoms of his/her disease. Poor health may lead to poor brain and organ functioning, and a quicker decline of healthy cells even before the transplant has begun. [4]

There are several ways in which one can optimize the health of their stem cells before and after stem cell collection and administration, respectively:

- Reduce sugar intake

- Reduce Triglycerides

- Reduce caloric intake

- Vitamins (especially C and D)

- Glucosamine and Chondroitin

- No steroids (avoid them) [5]

We have added a the end of the book an article about the importance of good nutrition, with some examples that may be interesting for the reader.

PHYSICAL ACTIVITY

A huge part of staying fit is getting up and moving around. Physical activity has been shown to affect each and every system of the body in different ways. Even a little bit of exercise stimulates the release of 'happy hormones' in the brain, hence mood is elevated.

It may be a surprise, but research shows that physical activity has an effect on muscle stem cells.

This is how it works; since exercise exerts a mechanical force on muscles, they sustain minor injuries in response to the strain. The injured tissue stimulates the production of stem cells in the muscle and accumulates there, post-exercise.

This collection of stem cells can serve as a stem-cell bank for the future, if needed. Stem cells consist of valuable anti-ageing properties. They can also be manipulated in a lab to yield specialized tissue cells, which can be used later for the therapy. Some of the common treated conditions are:

- Alzheimer's disease

- Spinal Cord Injury

- Stroke

- Heart disease

- Osteo-arthritis [6]

DETOXIFICATION THERAPY/CHELATION THERAPY

The objective of detoxification therapy is to get rid the body of free radicals and other harmful agents that have the ability to destroy healthy cells and tissues. This treatment involves the infusion of different vitamins, minerals, and the chemical substance EDTA. Heavy metals such as lead and mercury, and light metals such as calcium, bind to the agent and are excreted by the kidneys. EDTA stops the production of free radicals by eliminating the metal catalysts.

The other advantages of this process are:

- Excess calcium is also removed from the body

- Albumin bound calcium remains unaffected

- Bone calcium remains unaffected

- Reconditioning of cell function

What is detoxification used for?

Detoxification therapy is used for the following conditions:

- Diabetes mellitus

- Macular degeneration

- Arterial disease

- Multiple sclerosis

- Parkinson's disease

- Alzheimer's disease

The above-mentioned treatment regimens augment stem cell therapy by enhancing stem cells' health, and improving the overall fitness of the human body and mind. A healthy mind is a happy one!

REFERENCES

1. Elvis, A. M. (2011). Ozone therapy: A clinical review. Journal of Natural Science, Biology and Medicine, 66–70.

2. Kehr, W. (2016, October 3). Ozone Cancer Treatments. Retrieved from Cancer Tutor: https://www.cancertutor.com/ozone/

3. Latham, E. (2016, July 22). Hyperbaric oxygen therapy. Retrieved from Medscape: http://emedicine.medscape.com/article/1464149-overview

4. The Importance of Nutrition before Bone Marrow or Stem Cell Transplant. (2012). Retrieved from Bone Marrow Transplant at Angeles Health International: http://www.bonemarrowmx.com/the-importance-of-nutrition-before-bone-marrow-transplant-or-stem-cell-transplant/

5. Centeno, C. (2016, July 18). 8 Ways to increase stem cell health. Retrieved from Regennex: http://www.regenexx.com/8-ways-improve-your-stem-cells-prior-treatment/

6. Exercise triggers stem cells in muscle. (2012, February 6). Retrieved from Science Daily: https://www.sciencedaily.com/releases/2012/02/120206143944.htm

7. Tests and Procedures. Hyperbaric Oxygen Therapy. (1998-2016). Retrieved from Mayo Clinic: http://www.mayoclinic.org/tests-procedures/hyperbaric-oxygen-therapy/basics/why-its-done/prc-20019167

6

DIFFERENT APPROACHES OF MEDICINE

TRADITIONAL VS. ALTERNATIVE VS. HOMEOPATHIC MEDICINE

The word 'medicine' is an umbrella term. It encompasses much more than what it obviously states. Medicine is defined as "the science that deals with preventing, curing, and treating diseases" [1] or "a substance that is used in treating disease or relieving pain, and that is usually in the form of a pill or a liquid".

The first definition is more appropriate for the content of this chapter. This chapter will be describing the different phenomena by which the various forms of Medicine are used for healing purposes.

All different approaches of medicine enshrine a common goal, i.e. to achieve optimum health in an individual. They utilize different aspects of the human mind and body and incorporate them with their treatment formulas. The results vary from individual to individual. There are several factors that affect the outcome:

- Acute or chronic illness

- Local or systemic illness

- Co-morbid/ coexistent risk factors and/or illnesses

- One's belief (state of mind) in the treatment

The following are some of the different approaches of medicine; and how they differ from one another.

MAINSTREAM MEDICINE

Mainstream medicine is well-known and widely accepted as it is (more often than not) evidence-based. Case studies and research trials are carried out on a large scale and the results are published on highly authoritative platforms. The use of a pill, for instance, has become an everyday mode of treatment. It is not only easily accessible, but most of the pills are now available as over-the-counter drugs. The term itself implies that all other forms of medicine are outside mainstream or are unconventional. It is also known by other names such as western medicine, allopathic medicine, and orthodox medicine. [2]

Mainstream medicine has made groundbreaking leaps and bounds in the last couple of decades. One of the reasons is because the model to develop new drugs works. Let's start by having a group of people with a certain disease. This group gets organized and becomes a market. Then some entrepreneurs interested in the medicine field, invest in research together with universities and scientists. Once there are some signs of improving the health of this group, a pharmaceutical company gets involved taking the initial research to mature phases of clinical trials and secure patients for the formula. It takes a lot of time and money to develop a new drug, but once approved by the health department it goes into the target market. The whole process generates lots of income for the people involved and satisfies the need for those with that illness. So it's worthwhile and is a win-win situation. It is the name of a system in which Doctors and other health care providers treat the ill, using drugs, surgery, and radiation.

However, as with every system, there are downsides with this model. The main question that arises is what if the clinical trials do not show any positive results? The money invested goes to waste. What if some people take advantage of the system? They will keep receiving money for research but will spend the resources on "administrative expenses" not leaving enough for the real thing.

The worst situation of all is that rare diseases do not pose as an interesting market to pharmaceutical companies, therefore, some groups do not get constant research on their specific illness, leaving few options for treatment and hence, have to jump to other medicine approaches.

In the marketplace, different forms of medicine compete with mainstream medicine. A lot of people are growing skeptical of certain typical medical treatments. Firstly, because there's usually a plethora of side effects, and secondly, it can really put a burden on your pocket. Resorting to more natural treatment regimens can save you from both of these downfalls. However, there is a dire need for a complete examination and evaluation of one's condition before making a decision.

Stem cell therapy is slowly falling into the mainstream medicine category as a form of biological medicine. This treatment method is revolutionary in the sense that it is as natural as it can get as stem cells are almost always native in nature. They are free of manipulation and incoherencies. They are mostly used as stimulators, for replacement of unhealthy cells, and for the development of new and healthy tissue. They may take a longer time to show potential results, but that's only because they have to go through the natural process of division and development.

ALTERNATIVE & COMPLEMENTARY MEDICINE

Alternative medicine comprises of healing techniques that may or may not complement mainstream medicine, but lie outside the realm of orthodox medicine itself. For instance, there is much talk of acupuncture being the next big thing in the treatment of joint pains, headaches, and back pain. There are also other energy-stimulating methods, such as reiki and magnetic field therapy, which aim at restoring health with a 'healing touch'.[3]

Both of these terms are used interchangeably. However, there is a slight difference between them.[4]

If a non-mainstream procedure is used along with a mainstream medicine for treatment, it is called *"Complementary Medicine"*.

If a non-mainstream procedure is used in place of a mainstream medicine for treatment, it is called *"Alternative Medicine"*.

There are several examples of complementary (alternative) medicine:

- Natural products

- Yoga/ tai-chi

- Chiropractic or osteopathic manipulation

- Massage

- Special diets

- Relaxation techniques

- Deep breathing exercises

Homeopathic Medicine

Homeopathic medicine refers to a more holistic and natural approach to treating the sick. Homeopathic products are made from natural sources, be it from vegetables, animals, or minerals. It is based on different principles, such as 'like cures like', minimum dose, and single remedy.

Like cures like: The term homeopathy is derived from Latin, which means 'like disease'. Homeopathic medicine is prescribed, based on how the individual expresses the symptoms of the disease as a whole. It doesn't focus on the specific disease, rather the totality of the illness. This homeopathic law was threaded into the fabric of medicine in the mid-1800s. Medicine was given to healthy individuals (called provers). The symptoms they developed as a result of taking the medicine provided a homeopathic picture for that remedy. [5]

Minimum dose: Although homeopathic medicine is all natural, it can cause side effects, if given in the maximum dosage or in the crude form. For example, a certain type of relapsing fever was treated with Peruvian bark back in the day. When given in full strength, the patient got better but developed certain side effects as well. Later, the dose was tapered down to the minimum. This showed long lasting recovery.

Single remedy: Most homeopathic practitioners believe in prescribing a single remedy at a time to evaluate the effects of medicine on a single illness rather than prescribing more than one at the same time and assessing overshadowing results.

Why certain people respond better to different forms of medicine?

Some people believe that different treatment modalities have a place with mainstream medicine whereas many don't. It really depends on one's circumstances and underlying condition. What works for one may not necessarily work for another, simply due to the severity and intricacy of the illness and other factors that may influence it.

This often causes a dilemma for a physician who is constantly bombarded by questions about alternative and/or complementary techniques. Explaining the whole concept to a patient who is confused and unsure, can be challenging. It is best to educate yourself about the different forms of treatment, and whether your condition is the best candidate for it or not.

The most important point of all is to consult the experts in the respective fields. There are a lot of quacks out there that may end up worsening your condition. Take second opinions, if you must and only resort to the mode of treatment that satisfies you as a whole. There is nothing wrong by choosing what works specifically for you. Nothing trumps a healthy mind and body. Be positive in whatever you choose!

REFERENCES

1.   Merriam-Webster. (n.d.). Retrieved from Merriam-Webster Dictionary: http://www.merriam-webster.com/dictionary/medicine

2.   NCI Dictionary of Cancer Terms. (n.d.). Retrieved from National Cancer Institute: https://www.cancer.gov/publications/dictionaries/cancer-terms?cdrid=454747

3.   Complementary and Alternative Medicine (CAM). (2005-2016). Retrieved from WebMD: http://www.webmd.com/balance/what-is-alternative-medicine?page=2

4.   Complementary, Alternative, or Integrative Health: What's In a Name? (2016, June 28). Retrieved from National Centre for Complementary and Integrative Health: https://nccih.nih.gov/health/integrative-health

5.   What is Homeopathic Medicine? (2007-2016). Retrieved from American Institute of Homeopathy: http://homeopathyusa.org/homeopathic-medicine.html

7

INDICATIONS AND CONTRAINDICATIONS

FOR STEM CELL THERAPY

Some common questions when talking about stem cell therapy are: Who is the right patient? Am I a candidate for this kind of therapy? Who should not choose stem cell therapy for his condition? In the following paragraphs, we will try to answer all these questions.

Although stem cell therapy has made groundbreaking progress in the recent years, it has its limitations. Patients have to be evaluated thoroughly in order to categorize them as favorable or unfavorable candidates for the therapy. To weigh the alternatives, risks, and benefits of the procedure for the patient is an essential step prior to going through with any type of treatment. Stem cell therapy is as responsive as it is effective, therefore, all of its parameters have to be measured accurately to be on the safe side.

As stem cell infusion therapy promotes regeneration and self-healing, some consider it as an all-natural treatment for degenerative conditions of the body. It is ideal for patients in early stages of a disease, and also for people where autologous stem cell sources are a priority. For instance, those who are younger than 75 years old and want increased quality of life. It is ideal as a co-adjuvant of standard classic treatments.

Regeneration of body tissue is not a new concept and the use of stem cell therapy in mainstream medicine has been gaining worldwide acceptance. In recent years, advancements in molecular biology and biotechnology have become so fast paced that degenerative biological diseases are being treated with biology itself. It is really an astonishing principle.

Contraindications

There are certain conditions that are not recommended to be treated with stem cells as it would not result in a favorable outcome. For instance, if someone has one or several of the following, a deeper case study is recommended from your doctor to analyze other options with better outcome probabilities:

- Blood disorders

- Coagulation problems

- Anemia

- Concurrent bacterial infections

- Exaggerated vasculitis

- Acute thrombosis

- Expressed pulmonary hypertension secondary to vasculitis, thrombosis or pneumonia

- Myelofibrosis

- Terminal illness (intoxication, advanced metabolic syndrome, decompensation of internal organs

- Chronic infections

- Psychiatric diseases (risk of exacerbation)

- Cancer

There are other factors that also affect the effectiveness of stem cell therapy. The following factors are not contraindications but they decrease the possibility of obtaining full benefits from this kind of treatment:

- Age: Patient older than 75 years old, tend to have a slower response.

- Weight: It becomes highly invasive for young patients that weigh 30 kg or less, as it is aggressive, and harder to obtain autologous bone marrow from their bones or fat tissue from the abdominal area.

- Severity of disease: Stem cells work at their own pace, so a severely sick patient usually has a faster progression disease, therefore, not allowing the cells to distribute, engraft, grow, and heal.

It is worth mentioning that a positive attitude towards

healing helps your mind accept your current condition and automatically takes action of your everyday life increasing the possibilities of healing. A good attitude will help your state of mind, compelling you to practice good habits like healthy eating, physical activity, social life, etc. Happiness will follow you and every little improvement will be of value, will be taken positive and you will take advantage of such benefits. On the contrary, a negative attitude will most likely slow down your journey and make it more difficult along the way often resulting in depression and isolation. This attitude is usually accompanied by unreal expectations instead of realistic ones which make the task at hand i.e. to achieve a complete cure seem next to impossible.

Another key factor is the EXPECTATION that lags along with the patient. Although this is a natural thought and hopes to have, it has proven to be a definitive factor in deciding if one is the right patient for this therapy or not.

A very high expectation i.e. a complete "cure", makes you an unfavorable patient/candidate. Although stem cells have shown promising results and improvement, your body needs more than stem cells to get cured.

You are not a candidate if you expect a complete cure from stem cell therapy. For instance, Consider a 35-year-old male patient with renal failure who needs dialysis to maintain normal kidney function. The standard procedure probably is a kidney transplant. This patient is a bad candidate for stem cell therapy if he expects to avoid kidney transplant in the long run.

A low to mid expectation is a more practical and realistic approach on the matter in most cases. Stem cell therapy should be taken as a very good option/possibility of improvement for most conditions where it can help in reducing medications, increasing organ functions, and even postpone certain surgeries, etc. For instance, the 35-year-old patient with renal failure, could be considered as the perfect patient if his expectation is to improve his current health, improve his kidney function for months or even years. Meanwhile, a compatible kidney should be sought, so the transplant can be performed. Most likely his body will get to the transplant surgery in a better condition with previous stem cell therapy than without it, and as a consequence increase the probability of transplant success.

Proven Treatments vs. Syem Cell Therapy

If you have a condition where standard treatment has been proven to solve the problem, definitely we suggest for you to take the classic standard procedure. For example, cardiac valve surgery, hip replacements on a full wear bone, or antibiotic treatment for the acute phase of Lyme disease.

But, if your condition has treatment to control your health, but does not bring a solution, meaning you will have to take medication for life accepting side effects of such medication; then stem cell therapy can be very useful for you. For example, rheumatoid arthritis, multiple sclerosis, or diabetes.

Why? Because stem cell therapy is a biological treatment. It works differently in every person and in different degrees. So, a treatment where you can be sure that you will get cured is much more convenient, less time consuming, less expensive in the long run than a therapy still considered experimental in many instances. The opportunity of stem cell therapy should be taken even in conjunction with your current treatment, also, when your degenerative disease is not responding to standard procedure, and when cumulative side effects are a greater risk.

Although the list of conditions treated with stem cell therapy is big and every day more research adds new potential conditions that could be treated. The following are a few degenerative conditions that stem cell therapy had been used successfully, in chapter 8 we will go deeply on each one:

Indications for stem cell therapy:

Bone Disorders

- Osteoarthritis

- Osteogenesis imperfecta

- Non-healing fracture of bone

Osteoarthritis is a degenerative joint disease which comprises of mechanical abnormalities that are damaging the surrounding structures. Healing is not very common. The mainstream treatment comprises of pain relievers, supplements, and surgery in case of an unmanageable disease.

However, mesenchymal stem cells have been tested in bone disease, and the results have been promising. It promoted swifter healing. The stem cells could be obtained from bone marrow, harvested from the umbilical cord after birth, or from a fat mini-liposuction.

Immune Disorders

Stem cells not only have the ability to regenerate but they

can also modulate the immune system, thereby, halting any pathological responses by the immune system. [1]

A few examples are:

- Rheumatoid arthritis

- Scleroderma

- Lupus

Cardiovascular Disorders

- Heart failure

- Cardiomyopathy

- Acute Myocardial Infarction (MI)

Patients suffer most from acute cardiovascular injury. It is the negative reconstruction i.e. improper myocyte rebuilding and disorderly compensatory rebuilding that takes a toll on the ventricular function in the future.

Several clinical trials have been carried out to assess the efficacy of stem cell transplants in the setting of an acute Myocardial Infarction. Different stem cell types have been used with the aim of preserving the left ventricular function, to prevent the development of heart failure in the future.

However, much research still needs to be done on how to replace or regenerate dead myocytes surrounded by fibrous tissue. Stem cell therapy has not only opened doors for innovative treatment in the case of heart failure, but for the treatment of refractory angina pectoris, vascular insufficiency disorders, and chronic non-healing wounds as well. Although, research suggests efficacy, but the lack of specific guidelines limits the wide application of cell-based therapy in the setting of acute cardiovascular injury. [2]

Neurologic / Neuromuscular Disorders

- Parkinson's disease

- Alzheimer's disease

- Autism

- Cerebral Palsy

- Spinal Muscular atrophy

- Multiple sclerosis

- Stroke

Stem cell technology has been paving the way for better treatment options for neurodegenerative conditions like the ones mentioned above. The basic underlying problem is a loss of neurons in the brain or spinal cord. It may be acute as in stroke, or trauma, or it may be chronic as in Parkinson's and Alzheimer's. Cell-based therapy used for neuromuscular disorders has to be precisely based on the neuronal pathology of the disease as neurons carry out specific functions in specific parts of the brain. The focus of stem cell therapy here is either cellular replacement (as in Parkinson's disease in which a specific neuronal population is lost) or enriching the microenvironment (as in multiple sclerosis to support the remaining motor neurons).

Liver Disorders

LIVER CIRRHOSIS

The liver is well-known for its innate ability to regenerate. However, this is only advantageous when a certain portion of the liver is involved. Cirrhosis is a chronic condition in which the liver undergoes a process of 'scarring' or 'fibrosis' over a period of time. There are many underlying causes of a cirrhotic liver such as Hepatitis B and C, liver cancer, and biliary cirrhosis just to name a few. Cirrhosis causes irreversible damage to the liver and affects its ability to regenerate ultimately leading to liver failure. The only treatment of a cirrhotic liver is liver transplant which has in recent years gained popularity. Unfortunately, patients are forced to opt for other non-conventional treatment options due to lack of compatible organs, cost, lack of trained experts in this field, and go through other risks such as rejection. Statistics suggest that for every liver donor there are 30 recipients. Most succumb to liver failure while waiting.

Stem cell therapy has provided a beacon of hope to help such patients. Stem cell obtained from bone marrow, adipose tissue, and mesenchyme have the potential to differentiate into hepatocytes. Since they are harvested from the patient, there is no risk of rejection either. Besides regenerating, hepatocytes are also produced certain factors that promote regeneration and repair. Stem cell transplants have shown to be effective in treating degenerative liver conditions. [4]

Diabetes:

- Type I diabetes

- Type II diabetes

Diabetes is a condition in which the pancreas is dysfunctional in producing insulin (Type I) or insulin production is normal but the cells become resistant to the uptake of insulin (Type II). This results in high levels of blood glucose.

At present, the only treatment available for Type I diabetes is lifelong insulin injections and Type II is treated with medication, insulin, or a combination of both.

Stem cell therapy has a simple goal, i.e. to stimulate the cells to form pancreatic beta cells.[5,6] When technology evolves as such then we will be able to infuse them and control diabetes. Meanwhile, stem cells have shown to work well in conjunction with insulin administration. Although, there is no proof that stem cells produce pancreatic cells but they have shown a better control of blood glucose levels. Cases where insulin injections decreased from 4 to 2 a day. Cases where the body reacted positively where previous insulin rejection was found.

REFERENCES

1.   *Stem Cell Therapy* . (2016). Retrieved from Stem Cell Institute: https://www.
      cellmedicine.com/stem-cell-therapy-for-osteoarthritis/

2.   Behjati, M. (2013). Suggested indications of clinical practice guideline for
      stem cell-therapy in cardiovascular diseases: A stepwise appropriate use crite-
      ria for regeneration therapy. *ARYA Atherosclerosis* , 306-310.

3.   *Bone Marrow Aspiration and Biopsy*. (2015). Retrieved from Cancer.Net: http://
      www.cancer.net/navigating-cancer-care/diagnosing-cancer/tests-and-proce-
      dures/bone-marrow-aspiration-and-biopsy

4.   Centeno, C. (2016, July 18). *8 Ways to increase stem cell health*. Retrieved from
      Regennex: http://www.regenexx.com/8-ways-improve-your-stem-cells-prior-
      treatment/

5.   *Chronic liver disease: how could regenerative medicine help?* (2016). Retrieved from
      Swiss Medica: http://www.startstemcells.com/liver-cirrhosis-treatment.html

6.   *Diabetes: how could stem cells help?* (2015, November 09). Retrieved from Euro
      Stem Cell: http://www.eurostemcell.org/factsheet/diabetes-how-could-stem-
      cells-help

7.   Elvis, A. M. (2011). Ozone therapy: A clinical review. *Journal of Natural Science,
      Biology and Medicine* , 66-70.

8.   *Exercise triggers stem cells in muscle*. (2012, February 6). Retrieved from Science
      Daily: https://www.sciencedaily.com/releases/2012/02/120206143944.htm

9.   *Fat Stem Cell Therapy*. (2015). Retrieved from Infinite Horizons Medical Cen-
      ter: http://www.fatstemcelltherapy.com/procedure/

10.   Kehr, W. (2016, October 3). *Ozone Cancer Treatments*. Retrieved from Cancer
      Tutor: https://www.cancertutor.com/ozone/

11.   Latham, E. (2016, July 22). *Hyperbaric oxygen therapy*. Retrieved from Med-
      scape: http://emedicine.medscape.com/article/1464149-overview

12.   Lunn, J. S. (2011). Stem Cell Technology for Neurodegenerative Diseases.
       Ann Neurology , 353–361.

13.   Munoz J, S. N. (2014). umbilical cord blood transplantation: past, present,
       and future. *Stem Cells Transl Med* , 1435-1443.

14.   Patricia A. Zuk, *. M. (2002). Human Adipose Tissue Is a Source of Multipo-
       tent Stem Cells. *Molecular Biology of the Cell* , 4279–4295.

15.   *Stem cell harvest procedure.* (2016). Retrieved from Non Hodgkin Lymphoma
       Cyberfamily: http://www.nhlcyberfamily.org/treatments/collection.htm#-
       methods

16.   *Stem Cell Therapy* . (2016). Retrieved from Stem Cell Institute: https://www.
       cellmedicine.com/stem-cell-therapy-for-osteoarthritis/

17.   *Stem Cell Therapy and spinal cord injury.* (2016). Retrieved from Stem cell
       institute: https://www.cellmedicine.com/stem-cell-therapy-for-spinal-cord-
       injury/

18.   *Stem Cell/Bone Marrow Collection.* (n.d.). Retrieved from Blood and Marrow
       transplant information network: http://www.bmtinfonet.org/before/stem-
       cellmarrowharvest

19.   Terskikh AV, E. M. (2001). From hematopoiesis to neuropoiesis: evidence of
       overlapping genetic programs. *Proc Natl Acad Sci U S A* , 7934-9.

20.   *Tests and Procedures. Hyperbaric Oxygen Therapy.* (1998-2016). Retrieved from
       Mayo Clinic: http://www.mayoclinic.org/tests-procedures/hyperbaric-oxy-
       gen-therapy/basics/why-its-done/prc-20019167

21.   *The Bone Marrow Harvest Procedure.* (1995-2016). Retrieved from Cleveland
       Clinic: http://my.clevelandclinic.org/health/treatments_and_procedures/
       hic_Bone_Marrow_and_Transplantation/hic-bone-marrow-harvest-proce-
       dure

22.   *The Importance of Nutrition before Bone Marrow or Stem Cell Transplant.* (2012).
       Retrieved from Bone Marrow Transplant at Angeles Health International:
       http://www.bonemarrowmx.com/the-importance-of-nutrition-before-bone-
       marrow-transplant-or-stem-cell-transplant/

23.   *Turning Stem Cells into Insulin-Producing Cells.* (2016). Retrieved from Diabetes
       Research Institute Foundation: https://www.diabetesresearch.org/stem-cells

8

THERAPEUTIC USE OF STEM CELLS FOR DEGENERATIVE CONDITIONS

Degenerative disease is more of an umbrella term since it encompasses so many different conditions. They may have a different etiology, but the pathophysiology at the cellular level, remains the same i.e. it is a continuous process of cellular deterioration. Over the passage of time tissues and organs begin to wear and tear either due to natural processes, lifestyle choices (like exercise) and/or disease. (Motor Neuron Disease Information)

Unfortunately, degenerative conditions do not have a complete cure. In fact, the name indicates the disease process itself. With every passing day, the patient's status does not improve, rather it stays stagnant for some days while others may take a toll on the overall health. There are several factors like physical activity, diet, stress and psychology that play a role in the disease progression. Either way, the condition usually either stays the same or starts worsening with these external or internal factors. Medicines only help cope with some of the distressing symptoms.

A person suffering from a degenerative condition such as rheumatoid arthritis is most likely to experience intermittent attacks. In this case, bouts of joint pain and joint stiffness and immobility come and go. It is an inevitable and repetitive process. Depending on the symptoms, treatment aims to improve the quality of life and alleviate distress. Medications /drugs used to treat these kinds of conditions are common and easily accessible. However, they are not prescribed as a cure, but keep the symptoms under control and make life for the patient easier.

Having said this, there is a downside to consuming all these medications, i.e., they are usually needed for years and years until a new drug hits the market. Meanwhile, the patient usually ends up suffering from the side effects of these drugs, compromising the liver, kidney and even hurt in the long run. Due to lack of proper information and awareness, patients still prefer the long-term side effects as compared to the current treatment options for degenerative disease.

As stated above, the standard and well-known treatment for most degenerative conditions is medications/drugs. Most patients willingly opt for this option (and understandably so) as they have been researched, validated, and marketed for consumer use after relative authorization rendering them safe to use plus most of the times are paid by insurance. Now choosing to accept the standard treatment regimen means taking on the whole list of adverse effects the medications may cause as well. But, because the symptoms can become so debilitating at times, this part of the bargain is quite often overlooked.

This chapter will not focus on an opinion, rather research-based factual information on the basis of which anyone can make an informed decision about his/her health. It is worth mentioning here that patients who have opted for stem cell therapy to aid their degenerative conditions have not only shown an improved quality of life, but have recovered from the adverse effects and halted further organ damage by the medicines. One way or the other, the sooner the patient is treated with stem cell therapy the less damage he/she will have, which in turn ensures a better and faster regenerative response of stem cells. Hence, it is recommended to take action as soon as possible before further harm ensues.

Degenerative diseases can broadly be classified into 5 types:

1. Neurological conditions

2. Immunological conditions

3. Ophthalmologic conditions

4. Orthopedic conditions

5. Metabolic conditions

In the following section, we are going to describe the process of stem cell therapy for the above categories of degenerative conditions, it is important to mention that they are not the only ones that can benefit from stem cell therapy and since this is a science, it evolves continuously:

NEUROLOGIC CONDITIONS

MULTIPLE SCLEROSIS

OVERVIEW:

Multiple sclerosis (MS) is a condition of the central nervous system, which is known for its notoriousness. It can be benign in nature where the effects are negligible or it can progress to a debilitating extent.

CAUSE:

MS is thought to stem from an autoimmune etiology in which the body's own immune cells attack the myelin sheath that surrounds the nerves. This results in the disruption of various connections between the brain and other parts of the body. The exact trigger is unknown, however, it has been postulated that certain environmental factors may be responsible for the disease such as viruses. For example, Epstein Barr Virus (EBV) and Herpes Virus.[1]

SYMPTOMS:

The initial symptoms are blurred vision, red-green color distortions or blindness in one eye. More advanced symptoms include altered sensations in the limbs, paresthesia, 'pins and needles sensations', numbness, problems with coordination, etc. As the symptoms worsen, about half of MS patients experience cognitive impairment, poor judgment and memory which is often associated with depression. These generalized symptoms tend to be overlooked.

HOW STEM CELL THERAPY CAN HELP:

There has been ongoing research on the use of different types of stem cells for the treatment of MS and fortunately some cell types hold promise. Stem cells not only slow the progression of the disease, but can repair some of the damage done to the nerves as well.

Mesenchymal Stem cells are known for their ability to differentiate into any cell type. Several clinical trials are underway. For instance, phase 1 of a trial has been approved by the FDA, which has used mesenchymal stem cells for the treatment of MS. Mesenchymal stem cells have immune regulatory responses that can stop the body's immune cells from attacking the myelin sheaths. Mesenchymal stem cells may also have the potential to regenerate the myelin sheaths of the affected neurons.

Studies are being carried out at the Cambridge University on mesenchymal stem cells for the treatment of MS. [2]

Another type of stem cell that seems to be showing results in MS is the hematopoietic stem cell. MS therapy with these types of cells have shown a 70% success rate. A recent published study shows that HSCT could be the first MS therapy to reverse disability as it 'was associated with improvement in neurological disability and other clinical outcomes'. [3]

PATIENT PREPARATION

The patient is brought in for thorough evaluation prior to transplantation. The patient meets with a transplant expert who will review his/her medical record, discuss the treatment options and procedures, and will answer any questions that may come with.

If a patient is suffering from pain and inflammation, they will be administered respective medicines to relieve the symptoms before beginning therapy. A proper drug history is also very important as there are certain medicines that must be stopped at least a week before any procedure for example, blood thinners.

It is always a good idea for the body to be replenished continuously by nutrients like vitamins and minerals. Intravenous infusions or special diet may be recommended by a nutritionist or by your family doctor.

A simple psychological evaluation is carried out to see how the patient is dealing with stress and coping strategies. If there are psychological concerns a deeper evaluation is ordered.

STEM CELL SOURCE

In the case of MS, the use of mesenchymal stem cells has been advocated and supported through the evidence collected from clinical trials. Human mesenchymal stem cells are non-hematopoietic and possess the ability to differentiate into cells of mesodermal origin, such as osteocyte, chondrocytes and adipocytes; ectodermal origin, such as neurocytes and endodermal origin, such as hepatocytes. Mesenchymal stem cells are unique because they also consist of immune-modulatory characteristics, i.e. they can regulate the micro-environment in the host tissue. [4]

These cells are found in a variety of tissues such as:

• Bone marrow

• Adipose tissue

• Umbilical cord

Hematopoietic cells are also used from bone marrow. Allogenic stem cells are not recommended due to host-donor cell rejection or reaction. As described in chapter 4, usually the patient is given a local anesthetic and aspiration of bone marrow is performed.

STEM CELL PREPARATION

To ensure negligible damage to the stem cells, minimal manipulation of the bone marrow or source of mesenchymal stem cells is necessary. Cells are handled with care. Stem cells are not usually cryopreserved but they could be.

A specimen is divided in two parts: One part is usually combined with saline and other cell support reagents. While the second part is going to be concentrated; the red cells are removed, and some plasma is also removed. In this process all captured stem cells inside this components are spinned out into a buffer layer. This layer will be combined with a small volume of plasma obtaining a 1ml-3 ml concentrated dilution of stem cells.

STEM CELL INFUSION

For MS, the recommendation is to infuse part of the obtained specimen (mesenchymal stem cells) by IV route into the blood stream to regulate the immunological effects and with local anesthesia, the concentrated part of it infused by Intrathecal route to get into the spinal fluid to repair the myelin sheath around nerves. Mesenchymal stem cells have the potential to migrate into inflamed CNS tissue and express neuronal and glial cell markers. [5]

Hematopoietic stem cell therapy functions on 2 major principles in MS. One, as an immune-modulator as T-cells undergo a second phase of activation in this condition, hence, first-line immunomodulatory therapies in MS reduces the relapse rate and slow progression of disability. Secondly, some hematopoietic cells are recruited to sites of nerve damage to function as perivascular macrophage and microglia like cells. They can remove the cellular debris in the acute phase of injury.

SECONDARY EFFECTS AND RISKS

As mentioned in chapter 4, the side effects of a bone marrow aspiration are:

- Soreness and/or swelling in the following 3 days.

- For the intrathecal infusion there could be signs of soreness and redness. The risk involved in an intrathecal infusion is related to a bad positioning of the needle by an inexperienced doctor.

- A needle puncturing other tissues can produce inflammation, damage to nerves that can lead to other disabilities.

PARKINSON'S DISEASE

OVERVIEW:

Parkinson's disease is a neurological condition in which there is a gradual degeneration of neurons in the portion of the brain that controls movement. This disease usually has an adult onset, between the ages of 55-65. It is slightly more common in males than females.

CAUSE:

Parkinson's disease is caused primarily due to an imbalance of neurotransmitters in the basal ganglia (the portion of the brain that controls body movement). There are two main neurochemicals i.e. dopamine and acetylcholine that facilitate the transmission of nerve impulses. In this case, dopaminergic neurons begin to degenerate. Researchers believe there may be a genetic component as well. Very rarely is Parkinson's caused by viral infections or exposure to environmental toxins. Other causes of parkinsonism (read below) include:

- Adverse reaction to certain drugs

- Stroke

- Brain tumor

- Repeated head trauma

SYMPTOMS:

The primary symptoms of Parkinson's disease are stiffness, rigid and delayed movement (akinesia), mask like face, and resting tremors. Parkinson's disease is a form of parkinsonism which is a term that refers to a more generalized cluster of symptoms that may or may not occur in Parkinson's disease exclusively and may stem from other causes as well. More symptoms include:

- Impaired posture

- Slurred speech

- Loss of involuntary movements such as blinking and smiling

- Pill-rolling tremor; the back and forth movement of your thumb and forefinger

- Resting tremor; characteristic tremor in Parkinson's disease

HOW STEM CELL THERAPY CAN HELP:

Ongoing research has shown not only slow the progression of disease, but in some cases bringing to remission such progression. Even though there is no proof that stem cells are generating dopamine; they do promote or stimulate the activity of the remaining dopamine cell generators.

Mesenchymal Stem cells are known for their ability to differentiate into any cell type. Mesenchymal stem cells may have the potential to balance neurotransmitters in the basal ganglia and stimulate regeneration of remaining dopaminergic neurons, facilitating the transmission of nerve impulses. The key factor here is the word remaining, if the patient is treated sooner than later, there are more dopaminergic neurons that could be regenerated. Therefore, a patient with a well-advanced Parkinson, will have limited dopaminergic neurons available and will be harder expectation of recovery.

Hematopoietic stem cells seem to be showing improvements in patients with Parkinson's. These cells "run" around the body repairing organs and tissues, therefore creating a better overall health end environment that support the body, Even tissue of damaged cells as a consequence of the parkinsons, for example: adverse reaction of drugs or strokes.

A promising future includes various clinical trials and research with human umbilical cord matrix and umbilical cord blood where stem cells have been harvested and used in rats with Parrkinson's disease. The umbilical cord matrix and blood are sources rich in hematopoietic and mesenchymal stem cells. In addition to the large quantity, they are easy to harvest, it is cost effective, and they can be frozen for future use. These cells when injected into rats with Parrkinson's showed partial reversal of the Parkinsonian phenotype. [6]

Embryonic stem cells could become in the future also a common use in the treatment of Parkinson's disease to replace degenerating dopaminergic neurons. Embryonic cells differentiate into neuronal stem cells of the mid-brain (which is affected by Parkinson's) and exhibit the same electro-physiological and behavioral properties as expected of the neurons in the mid brain. [7]

PATIENT PREPARATION

The patient is brought in for thorough evaluation prior to transplantation. The patient meets with a transplant expert who will review his/her medical record, discuss the treatment options and procedures, and will answer any questions that may come with.

If a patient is suffering from tremors, pain and inflammation, they will be administered respective medicines to relieve the symptoms before beginning therapy. A proper drug history is also very important as there are certain medicines that must be stopped at least a week before any procedure for example, blood thinners. If tremors are severe some indications will have to be followed since there are moments during a medical procedure where no movement is need it, specially while bone marrow aspiration is performed.

It is always a good idea for the body to be replenished continuously by nutrients like vitamins and minerals. Intravenous infusions or special diet may be recommended by a nutritionist or by your family doctor.

A simple psychological evaluation is carried out to see how the patient is dealing with stress and coping strategies. If there are psychological concerns a deeper evaluation is ordered.

STEM CELL SOURCE

Autologous Hematopoietic cells are used for this condition. Usually harvested from bone marrow. As described in chapter 4, usually the patient is given a local anesthetic and aspiration of bone marrow without pain is performed.

Mesenchymal stem cells have also been advocated and

supported through the evidence collected from clinical trials. Therefore in some cases where the condition of the patient is appropriate adipose tissue is collected as described in chapter 4.

STEM CELL PREPARATION

To ensure negligible damage to the stem cells, minimal manipulation of the bone marrow stem cells is necessary. Cells are handled with care. Stem cells are not usually cryopreserved.

A specimen is divided in two parts: One part is usually combined with saline and other cell support reagents. While the second part is going to be concentrated; the red cells are removed, and some plasma is also removed. In this process all captured stem cells inside this components are spinned out into a buffer layer. This layer will be combined with a small volume of plasma obtaining a 1ml-3 ml concentrated dilution of stem cells.

STEM CELL INFUSION

For Parkinson's disease (PD), the recommendation is to infuse part of the obtained specimen by I.V. into the blood stream, it will regulate some of the effects of the condition. Also with some local anesthesia help, the concentrated part mentioned above is infused by an Intrathecal injection to get stem cells into the spinal fluid. This high dose of stem cells have the potential to migrate and slow down or even stop degeneration of nigrostriatal dopaminergic neurons.

The grafted stem cells help neurons survive and regenerate new neurons in the striatum for as long as 10 years, despite an ongoing disease process, which destroys the patient's own dopaminergic neurons. The grafts are able to function as normal striatal dopaminergic neurons. They have also shown to reverse the underlying akinesia. Some patients lower or withdraw from L-dopa treatment for several years and resume a better quality of life.

SECONDARY EFFECTS AND RISKS

As mentioned in chapter 4, the side effects of a bone marrow aspiration are:

- Soreness and/or swelling in the following 3 days.

- For the intrathecal infusion there could be signs of soreness and redness. The risk involved in an intrathecal infusion is related to a bad positioning of the needle by and inexperienced doctor.

- A needle puncturing other tissues can produce inflammation, damage to nerves that can lead to other disabilities.

ALZHEIMER'S DISEASE

OVERVIEW:

Alzheimer's disease is a progressive neurodegenerative disorder which is characterized by dementia or memory loss. There could be episodic or semantic memory loss along with impairment of intellect. Alzheimer's disease makes up about 60-80% of dementia cases.

CAUSE:

The etiology of Alzheimer's disease for the most part is genetic in nature. It is thought to arise from a genetic mutation. Other causes include certain environmental factors, toxins and lifestyle. The cholinergic neurons of the basal forebrain are primarily affected by AD. Microscopic examination reveals the deposition of intracellular and extracellular β- amyloid or Abeta (Aβ) protein, intracellular formation of neurofibrillary tangles and neuronal loss.

SYMPTOMS:

- Repetitive questions and/or conversations

- Misplacing personal belongings

- Getting lost on a familiar route

- Decision-making skills lessen with time

- Poor judgment

- Unable to manage finances

- Inability to recognize common faces

- Spelling or writing errors

- Change in personality or behavior

HOW CAN STEM CELL THERAPY HELP?

Stem cell therapy may become the mainstream treatment for neurodegenerative diseases like Alzheimer's. As mentioned earlier, the cholinergic neurons of the basal forebrain are damaged in this condition. Clinical studies have shown that grafted neural precursor stem cells have shown incorporation into the surrounding parenchyma and have also exhibited differentiation into functional neural lineages. The advantages don't end here. The stem cells not only replace the damaged neurons, but also stimulate endogenous neural precursors, enhance the structure of the microenvironment and reduce pro-inflammatory cytokines in the affected area. [8]

PATIENT PREPARATION

The patient is brought in for thorough evaluation prior to transplantation. The patient meets with a transplant expert who will review his/her medical record, discuss the treatment options and procedures, and will answer any questions that may come with.

If a patient is suffering from pain and inflammation, they will be administered respective medicines to relieve the symptoms before beginning therapy. A proper drug history is also very important as there are certain medicines that must be stopped at least a week before any procedure for example, blood thinners.

It is always a good idea for the body to be replenished continuously by nutrients like vitamins and minerals. Intravenous infusions or special diet may be recommended by a nutritionist or by your family doctor.

A simple psychological evaluation is carried out to see how the patient is dealing with stress and coping strategies. If there are psychological concerns a deeper evaluation is ordered.

STEM CELL SOURCE

Stem cells for Alzheimer's are usually harvested from bone marrow therefore will be a combination of Autologous Hematopoietic cells and Mesenchymal stem cells. As described in chapter 4, usually the patient is given a local anesthetic and aspiration of bone marrow without pain is performed.

In some cases, where the health of the patient is adequate, adipose tissue could also be collected as described in chapter 4. The adipose tissue is rich on mesenchymal stem cells , they are multipotent in nature and hence can differentiate into any cell type. These cells have also been advocated and supported through the evidence collected from clinical trials.

STEM CELL PREPARATION

To ensure negligible damage to the stem cells, minimal manipulation of the bone marrow stem cells is necessary. Cells are handled with care. Stem cells are not usually cryopreserved.

A specimen is divided in two parts: One part is usually combined with saline and other cell support reagents. While the second part is going to be concentrated; the red cells are removed, and some plasma is also removed. In this process all captured stem cells inside this components are spinned out into a buffer layer. This layer will be combined with a small volume of plasma obtaining a 1ml-3 ml concentrated dilution of stem cells.

STEM CELL INFUSION

Neural precursor stem cells are divided in 2 parts. Part one is infused by IV into the blood stream, they will regulate some of the effects of the condition. And part 2, the concentrated part mentioned above, is infused by an Intrathecal injection. The goal is to get stem cells into the spinal fluid. The intrathecal injection is performed with local anesthesia to eliminate any discomfort.

Both parts, the stem cells exhibit targeted migration towards the damaged regions of the brain where they mature and proliferate into mature neurons. This results in improvement of learning and retention deficits.

SECONDARY EFFECTS AND RISKS:

As mentioned in chapter 4, the side effects of a bone marrow aspiration are:

•   Soreness and/or swelling in the following 3 days.

For the intrathecal infusion there could be signs of soreness and redness. The risk involved in an intrathecal infusion is related to a bad positioning of the needle by and inexperienced doctor.

- A needle puncturing other tissues can produce inflammation, damage to nerves that can lead to other disabilities.

AMYOTROPHIC LATERAL SCLEROSIS

OVERVIEW:

Amyotrophic Lateral Sclerosis (ALS) is a progressive neurological disorder that affects the neurons responsible for controlling voluntary muscles of the body also known as motor neurons. ALS is part of a group of disorders called Motor Neuron Disease. Such disorders exhibit a progressive degeneration of both upper and lower motor neurons. Upper motor neurons connect the brain to the spinal cord and lower motor neurons relay signals from the spinal cord to the respective muscles of the body.

CAUSE:

- About 5-10% of cases are familial i.e. they are inherited. One parent who carries a gene for ALS is enough to pass it on to the next generation. Familial ALS is caused by mutations in more than a dozen genes.

- About 90% of ALS cases are sporadic i.e. with random occurrence, no family history or apparent cause.

- Males are slightly more at risk to develop ALS than females.

- Age prevalence is 55-75 years.

SYMPTOMS:

- Fasciculation or muscle twitches

- Muscle spasticity

- Muscle atrophy

- Slurred speech

- Difficulty in swallowing/chewing

Some may experience the initial symptoms in the hand, arm or leg and find difficulty in specialized tasks like buttoning a shirt, writing or repetitive stumbling on walking. This is known as 'limb onset' ALS. Others may have trouble in swallowing or chewing hence termed as 'Bulbar onset' ALS. [9]

HOW CAN STEM CELL THERAPY HELP:

ALS is a progressive neurodegenerative condition that can be fatal as it expands to the respiratory stage. Currently, antioxidants and infusion of trophic molecules are being used to treat this disease.

A clinical study was carried out on 9 patients with definitive ALS. Autologous mesenchymal stem cells were harvested from their bone marrow and transplanted. These patients were observed over a period of 4 years and results suggested that there was a significant decline in the progression of disease in 4 of the 9 patients. [10]

Proper expectation must be understood by the patients in any case, but most important on ALS cases. In our experience we have seen benefits such as slowing the progression of the disease, an overall increase of organ function and better blood tests. Even though stopping the progression is the main goal, we have not seen such response.

PATIENT PREPARATION

The patient is brought in for thorough evaluation prior to procedure. The patient meets with the medical team who will review his/her medical record, discuss the treatment options and procedures, and will answer any questions that may come with.

If a patient is suffering from pain and inflammation, they will be administered respective medicines to relieve the symptoms before beginning therapy. If any infection is detected, it will be treated with the standard protocol and the stem cell procedure will be postponed. A proper drug history is also very important as there are certain medicines that must be stopped at least a week before any procedure for example, blood thinners.

It is always a good idea for the body to be replenished continuously by nutrients like vitamins and minerals. Intravenous infusions or special diet may be recommended by a nutritionist or by your family doctor.

A simple psychological evaluation is carried out to see how the patient is dealing with stress and coping strategies. If there are psychological concerns a deeper evaluation is ordered.

STEM CELL SOURCE

Autologous stem cells are a good source of stem cell therapy for ALS as there is minimal risk of rejection/reaction. Allogeneic stem cells, undifferentiated or transdifferentiated and manipulated epigenetically or genetically, could also be used for local or systemic cell-therapies in ALS. [11]

Taking into consideration that ALS is a very aggressive and fast-paced disease, our best course of action is to defend the body with the most stem cells available and the most amount of them possible. By using a combination of Bone marrow stem cells, Adipose tissue stem cells and placental/umbilical cord stem cells we create a high concentrated stem cell enviroment with many different kind of subsets of cells and therefore we expect a faster engraftment, a more efficient cell expansion and ultimately outpace the aggressiveness of the disease.

STEM CELL PREPARATION

To ensure negligible damage to the stem cells, minimal manipulation of the bone marrow stem cells is considered. Cells are handled with care and freshness is preferred over cryopreservation.

Adipose tissue is processed in the lab following the highest standards, stem cells are separated from fat and put into expansion for a few weeks. Once a large specimen is ready is harvested from culture flasks and prepared into a syrenge ready for infusion.

Umbilical cord stem cells usually are frozen in a tissue bank. After being received, they pass through a process of validation to make sure they are safe to use. Validation of infectious disease and verification of patient compatibility. Then they are thawed from their cryopreservation stage, cryopreservation protectant is washed out and there are 2 options, either using them as they are, or putting them into culture to expand the number of them similar to adipose tissue.

Depending on the doctor treatment protocol: some cells will be prepared into an IV solution and some of them into a concentrated solution for direct injection.

STEM CELL INFUSION

When using different kind of stem cells sources we make sure they are not combined into one big solution. There will be several infusions one for each kind of stem cell source, and most likely separated by several hours, they are even separated 24 hrs between them.

Intravenous drip of stem cell solution coming from an individual source into the blood stream will regulate the immunological effects and help with the overall regeneration of the internal organs.

Also, with local anesthesia, the concentrated stem cells are injected by Intrathecal route to get into the spinal fluid. The spinal fluid with its natural flow transport the stem cells and washes the brain. The interaction of the stimulous of the stem cells increases neurological connections and improves efficency of internal communication facilitiating the neurons generative process.

NEUROLOGIC CONDITIONS   129

SECONDARY EFFECTS AND RISKS

As mentioned in chapter 4, the side effects of a bone marrow aspiration are:

- Soreness and/or swelling in the following 3 days.

- For the intrathecal infusion there could be signs of soreness and redness.   The risk involved in an intrathecal infusion is related to a bad positioning of the needle by and inexperienced doctor.

- A needle puncturing other tissues can produce inflammation, damage to nerves that can lead to other disabilities.

- Cord blood stem cells if not HLA compatible could cause an immuno rejection, a allergic reactions that could lead to very serious complications. Depending on the severity of the reactions, patients' lives can be compromised.

AUTISM

OVERVIEW:

Autism is a neurological as well as a developmental disorder, hence the symptoms occur early on in childhood and last for a lifetime. It is now referred to as Autism Spectrum Disorder as people who suffer from it manifest a range of symptoms. Such people will often differ in their mannerisms in learning, communicating, and interacting with others.

CAUSE:

The exact cause of ASD is unknown, however there is a theory which states it is a genetic condition. Another theory postulates that it may be associated with autoimmune disease related or unrelated to vaccines. In either case, neurophysiological and neural hypo-perfusion abnormalities are a constant. There are certain environmental factors, diet and lifestyle factors that may aggravate or ameliorate the condition.

SYMPTOMS:

The cognitive condition may vary from extremely gifted to severely challenged. Since there is such a wide range of symptoms, it is either very easily overlooked or over-diagnosed.

Here are some symptoms to look out for in the early years of development: [12]

- Not responding to name by 12 months of age

- Avoids eye contact

- Unable to socialize

- Delayed speech and language skills

- Repetition of words and phrases

- Gives unrelated answers to questions

- Gets upset with minor changes in routine

- Flaps hands or spins in circles

   Symptoms associated with social skills may be:

- Avoids eye contact

- Prefers to play alone

- Expressionless face

- Does not share interests with others

- Does not understand personal space and boundaries

- Difficult to console during stress

- Has trouble understanding other people's feelings and communicating own feelings

HOW CAN STEM CELL THERAPY HELP:

Recent studies suggest that ASD may be associated with autoimmune disorders. Stem cell therapy has been used for a variety of autoimmune conditions, such as Sclerodermia, Lupus or Crohn's disease. As mentioned above, stem cells comprise of immune modulating properties and have been used in about 10 clinical trials for ASD treatment. Some patients have shown benefit from treatment but more scientific evidence needs to be collected.

As mentioned above, ASD stems from dysfunctional neurons, a decreased blood supply to the affected area of the brain and auto-immune process. Stem cells can help in all three areas as the combination of hematopoietic and mesenchymal stem cells could stimulate the formation of functional neurons, increase blood flow by formation of new vessels and control the autoimmune process.

PATIENT PREPARATION

The patient is brought in for thorough evaluation prior to transplantation. The patient meets with a transplant expert who will review his/her medical record, discuss the treatment options and procedures, and will answer any questions that may come with.

In addition a psychological evaluation is carried out by a neurologist to see how the patient is dealing with daily activities and qualifiy as a candidate for this kind of therapy. If there are psychological concerns a deeper evaluation is ordered.

If a patient is suffering from pain and inflammation, they will be administered respective medicines to relieve the symptoms before beginning therapy. A proper drug history is also very important as there are certain medicines that must be stopped at least a week before any procedure for example, blood thinners.

It is always a good idea for the body to be replenished continuously by nutrients like vitamins and minerals. Intravenous infusions or special diet may be recommended by a nutritionist or by your family doctor.

STEM CELL SOURCE

In the case of Autism, the use of bone marrow as a source of hematopoietic and mesenchymal stem cells has been supported through the evidence collected from research and clinical trials. These stem cells possess the ability to differentiate into cells of ectodermal origin, such as neurocytes and they also consist of immune-modulatory characteristics, i.e. they can regulate the micro-environment in the host tissue.[4]

Another good source of stem cells is the adipose tissue. Since most of patients with autism are children, we do not recommend performing a mini-liposuction in children. It is very aggressive, the fat layer is thin and risks are higher, therefore adipose tissue is not a preferred source.

Hematopoietic cells are commonly harvested from bone marrow. Allogenic stem cells are not recommended due to host-donor cell rejection or reaction. As described in chapter 4, usually the patient is given a local anesthetic and aspiration of bone marrow is performed.

If the patient had stored stem cells from the umbilical cord blood when he was born, then it could be a viable source of stem cells for this type of condition.

STEM CELL PREPARATION

To ensure negligible damage to the stem cells, minimal manipulation of the bone marrow is necessary. Cells are handled with care. Stem cells are not usually cryopreserved but they could be.

A specimen is divided in two parts: One part is usually combined with saline and other cell support reagents. While the second part is going to be concentrated; the red cells are removed, and some plasma is also removed. In this process all captured stem cells inside these components are spinned out into a buffer layer. This layer will be combined with a small volume of plasma obtaining a 1ml-3 ml concentrated dilution of stem cells.

STEM CELL INFUSION

Since most of the cases of Autism are children, and they are easily scared by needles, a light sedation is recommended. Patient is asked to be early morning at the procedure room before any meal. Fasting will enable better tolerance to light anesthesia.

After the patient is sedated, an IV will be set and then the procedure of bone marrow aspiration begins.

The best results had been obtained when one part of the specimen is infused by IV into the blood stream to regulate the immunological effects and the concentrated part of it infused by Intrathecal route to get into the spinal fluid to flow up to the brain and stimulate the brain barrier and neurons.

SECONDARY EFFECTS AND RISKS

As mentioned in chapter 4, the side effects of a bone marrow aspiration are:

- Soreness and/or swelling in the following 3 days.

- For the intrathecal infusion there could be signs of soreness and redness. The risk involved in an intrathecal infusion is related to a bad positioning of the needle by and inexperienced doctor.

- A needle puncturing other tissues can produce inflammation, damage to nerves that can lead to other disabilities.

Besides the common side effects of an IV and the intrathecal infusion, there are also side effects from the light general anesthesia or Sedation:

- Children can have a reaction to the anesthesia

- After the procedure, the patient can experience confusion, nausea and dizziness.

- Patient will be tired and could sleep for many hours after the procedure.

STROKE AND TRAUMATIC BRAIN INJURY

OVERVIEW:

A stroke and traumatic brain injury are more common than one may think. For instance, they are both acute injuries and both result in functional impairment depending upon the part of the brain affected. The symptomatology and etiology may differ.

CAUSE:

Causes of stroke:

- Obesity

- Alcohol

- Physical inactivity

- Hypercholesterolemia

- Diabetes

- Sleep apnea

Causes of TBI:

- Top 3 causes of TBI are car accidents, firearms and falls.

- Chemical/Toxic injury

- Hypoxic (lack of oxygen) injury

- Tumors

- Infections

- Stroke

SYMPTOMS:

- Confusion

- Disorientation

- Paralysis of limb(s)

- Trouble with speaking and understanding

- Visual impairment

- Headache (persistent and gets worse with time) [14]

- Convulsions or seizures

- Slurred or incoherent speech

HOW STEM CELL THERAPY CAN HELP?

Stroke is a phenomenon in which lack of blood flow causes ischemic injury not only to the neurons, but surrounding cells in the brain parenchyma as well like glial and endothelial cells. Transplanting stem cells directly to the affected area of the cerebrum will not only form new, functional neurons but also stimulate angiogenesis. Research suggests that stem cell therapy promotes endogenous repair mechanisms and reduces cell death.[15]

Several clinical studies suggests that the infusion on neural stem cell precursors and direct implant of neural stem cells showed improvement in motor function. However, more evidence is needed to deduce the effects on other functions.

PATIENT PREPARATION

The patient is brought in for thorough evaluation prior to transplantation. The patient meets with a transplant expert who will review his/her medical record, discuss the treatment options and procedures, and will answer any questions that may come with.

It is always a good idea for the body to be replenished continuously by nutrients like vitamins and minerals. Intravenous infusions or special diet may be recommended by a nutritionist or by your family doctor.

A psychological evaluation is carried out to see how the patient is dealing with daily activities. If there are psychological concerns a deeper evaluation is ordered.

STEM CELL SOURCE

Stem cells for TBI or Stroke are usually harvested from bone marrow therefore will be a combination of Autologous Hematopoietic cells and Mesenchymal stem cells. As described in chapter 4, usually the patient is given a local anesthetic and aspiration of bone marrow without pain is performed.

In some cases, where the health of the patient is adequate, adipose tissue could also be collected as described in chapter 4. The adipose tissue is rich on mesenchymal stem cells, they are multipotent in nature and hence can differentiate into any cell type. These cells have also been advocated and supported through the evidence collected from clinical trials.

STEM CELL PREPARATION

In order to ensure negligible damage to the stem cells, minimal manipulation of the bone marrow stem cells is necessary. Cells are handled with care. Stem cells are not usually cryopreserved.

Specimen is divided in two parts: One part is usually combined with saline and other cell support reagents. While the second part is going to be concentrated; the red cells are removed, and some plasma is also removed. In this process all captured stem cells inside this components are spinned out into a buffer layer. This layer will be combined with a small volume of plasma obtaining a 1ml-3 ml concentrated dilution of stem cells.

STEM CELL INFUSION

Neural precursor stem cells are divided in 2 parts. Part one is infused by I.V. into the blood stream, they will regenerate damaged cells and tissues, also will increase efficiency of internal organs. And part 2, the concentrated part mentioned above, is infused by an Intrathecal injection. The goal is to get stem cells into the spinal fluid. The intrathecal injection is performed with local anesthesia to eliminate any discomfort.

Both parts, the stem cells exhibit targeted migration towards the damaged regions of the brain where they mature and proliferate into mature neurons. Also they will have an effect of better communication between neurons by creating new connections between them. Resulting in improvement of brain function, thus increasing physical mobility, sensibility, reasoning, attention, focus, etc.

SECONDARY EFFECTS AND RISKS:

As mentioned in chapter 4, the side effects of a bone marrow aspiration are:

- Soreness and/or swelling in the following 3 days.

For the intrathecal infusion there could be signs of soreness and redness. The risk involved in an intrathecal infusion is related to a bad positioning of the needle by and inexperienced doctor.

- A needle puncturing other tissues can produce inflammation, damage to nerves that can lead to other disabilities.

REFERENCES

1.   Martin R, M. H. (January 24, 2017). Assessment of Patients With Multiple Sclerosis (MS). *National Institute of Neurological Disorders and Stroke (NINDS)*.

2.   Riordan, N. (2016). *Stem Cell Therapy* . Retrieved from stem cell Institute: https://www.cellmedicine.com/stem-cell-therapy-for-multiple-sclerosis-3/

3.   Richard K. Burt, M., Roumen Balabanov, M., Xiaoqiang Han, M., & al, e. (2015). Association of Nonmyeloablative Hematopoietic Stem Cell Transplantation With Neurological Disability in Patients With Relapsing-Remitting Multiple Sclerosis. *Journal of the American Medical Association (JAMA).* , 275-284.

4.   Imran Ullah, *. R. (2015). Human mesenchymal stem cells - current trends and future prospective. *Bioscience Reports*, 35 (2)

5.   Iajimi, A. A. (2013). Feasibility of Cell Therapy in Multiple Sclerosis: A Sys-
      tematic Review of 83 Studies. *International Journal of Hematology-Oncology and
      Stem Cell Research*, 15-33.

6.   Weiss, M. L. (2005). Human Umbilical Cord Matrix Stem Cells: Prelimi-
      nary Characterization and Effect of Transplantation in a Rodent Model of
      Parkinson's Disease. *Stem Cells*.

7.   Kim, J.-H. (2002). Dopamine neurons derived from embryonic stem cells
      function in an animal model of Parkinson's disease. *nature, International weekly
      journal of Science*, 50-56.

8.   OM, A.-S. (2011). Stem cell therapy for Alzheimer's disease. *CNS Neurological
      DIsroders Drug Targets*, 459-85

9.   *ALS Fact Sheet*. (n.d.). Retrieved from National Institute of Neurological Dis-
      orders and Stroke: https://www.ninds.nih.gov/Disorders/Patient-Caregiv-
      er-Education/Fact-Sheets/Amyotrophic-Lateral-Sclerosis-ALS-Fact-Sheet

10.   Mazzini, L. (2008). Stem cell treatment in Amyotrophic Lateral Sclerosis.
      Journal of the Neurological Sciences, 78–83.

11.   Prof Vincenzo Silani, M. (2004). Stem-cell therapy for amyotrophic lateral
      sclerosis. *The Lancet*, 200–202.

12.   *Signs and Symptoms of ASD*. (n.d.). Retrieved from Centres for Disease Control
      and Prevention: https://www.cdc.gov/ncbddd/autism/signs.html

13.   Ichim, T. E. (2007). Stem Cell Therapy for Autism. *Journal of Translational
      Medicine*, 5:30.

14.   *Traumatic Brain Injury*. (2016, October 11). Retrieved from Medline Plus:
      https://medlineplus.gov/traumaticbraininjury.html#cat95

15.   *ALS Fact Sheet*. (n.d.). Retrieved from National Institute of Neurological Dis-
      orders and Stroke: https://www.ninds.nih.gov/Disorders/Patient-Caregiv-
      er-Education/Fact-Sheets/Amyotrophic-Lateral-Sclerosis-ALS-Fact-Sheet

16.   Ballabio, F. L. (2009). Stem cell therapy in stroke. *Cellular and Molecular Life
      Sciences* , 757–772.

17.   Behjati, M. (2013). Suggested indications of clinical practice guideline for
      stem cell-therapy in cardiovascular diseases: A stepwise appropriate use crite-
      ria for regeneration therapy. *ARYA Atherosclerosis* , 306-310.

18.   *Bone Marrow Aspiration and Biopsy.* (2015). Retrieved from Cancer.Net: http://www.cancer.net/navigating-cancer-care/diagnosing-cancer/tests-and-procedures/bone-marrow-aspiration-and-biopsy

19.   Centeno, C. (2016, July 18). *8 Ways to increase stem cell health.* Retrieved from Regennex: http://www.regenexx.com/8-ways-improve-your-stem-cells-prior-treatment/

20.   *Chronic liver disease: how could regenerative medicine help?* (2016). Retrieved from Swiss Medica: http://www.startstemcells.com/liver-cirrhosis-treatment.html

21.   *Diabetes: how could stem cells help?* (2015, November 09). Retrieved from Euro Stem Cell: http://www.eurostemcell.org/factsheet/diabetes-how-could-stem-cells-help

22.   Elvis, A. M. (2011). Ozone therapy: A clinical review. *Journal of Natural Science, Biology and Medicine* , 66–70.

23.   *Exercise triggers stem cells in muscle.* (2012, February 6). Retrieved from Science Daily: https://www.sciencedaily.com/releases/2012/02/120206143944.htm

24.   *Fat Stem Cell Therapy.* (2015). Retrieved from Infinite Horizons Medical Center: http://www.fatstemcelltherapy.com/procedure/

25.   Ichim, T. E. (2007). Stem Cell Therapy for Autism. *Journal of Translational Medicine* , 5:30.

26.   Imran Ullah, *. R. (2015). Human mesenchymal stem cells - current trends and future prospective. *Bioscience Reports* , 35 (2).

27.   Kehr, W. (2016, October 3). *Ozone Cancer Treatments.* Retrieved from Cancer Tutor: https://www.cancertutor.com/ozone/

28.   Kim, J.-H. (2002). Dopamine neurons derived from embryonic stem cells function in an animal model of Parkinson's disease. *nature, International weekly journal of Science* , 50-56.

29.   lajimi, A. A. (2013). Feasibility of Cell Therapy in Multiple Sclerosis: A Systematic Review of 83 Studies. *International Journal of Hematology-Oncology and Stem Cell Research* , 15-33.

30.   Latham, E. (2016, July 22). *Hyperbaric oxygen therapy.* Retrieved from Medscape: http://emedicine.medscape.com/article/1464149-overview

31.   Lunn, J. S. (2011). Stem Cell Technology for Neurodegenerative Diseases. *Ann Neurology* , 353–361.

32.   Martin R, M. H. (January 24, 2017). Assessment of Patients With Multiple
       Sclerosis (MS). *National Institute of Neurological Disorders and Stroke (NINDS)* .

33.   Mazzini, L. (2008). Stem cell treatment in Amyotrophic Lateral Sclerosis.
       Journal of the Neurological Sciences , 78–83.

34.   McKhann GM, K. D. (2011). The diagnosis of dementia due to Alzheimer's
       disease: Recommendations from the National Institute on Aging-Alzheimer's
       Association workgroups on diagnostic guidelines for Alzheimer's disease.
       Alzheimer's and Dementia , 263-269.

35.   *Motor Neuron Disease Information.* (n.d.). Retrieved from National Institute of
       Neurological Diseases and Stroke: https://www.ninds.nih.gov/Disorders/
       All-Disorders/Motor-Neuron-Diseases-Information-Page

36.   Munoz J, S. N. (2014). umbilical cord blood transplantation: past, present,
       and future. *Stem Cells Transl Med* , 1435-1443.

37.   OM, A.-S. (2011). Stem cell therapy for Alzheimer's disease. *CNS Neurological
       DIsroders Drug Targets* , 459-85.

38.   Patricia A. Zuk, *. M. (2002). Human Adipose Tissue Is a Source of Multipo-
       tent Stem Cells. *Molecular Biology of the Cell* , 4279–4295.

39.   Prof Vincenzo Silani, M. (2004). Stem-cell therapy for amyotrophic lateral
       sclerosis. *The Lancet* , 200–202.

40.   Richard K. Burt, M., Roumen Balabanov, M., Xiaoqiang Han, M., & al, e.
       (2015). Association of Nonmyeloablative Hematopoietic Stem Cell Trans-
       plantation With Neurological Disability in Patients With Relapsing-Remitting
       Multiple Sclerosis. *Journal of the American Medical Association (JAMA).* , 275-284.

41.   Riordan, N. (2016). *Stem Cell Therapy* . Retrieved from stem cell Institute:
       https://www.cellmedicine.com/stem-cell-therapy-for-multiple-sclerosis-3/

42.   *Signs and Symptoms of ASD.* (n.d.). Retrieved from Centres for Disease Control
       and Prevention: https://www.cdc.gov/ncbddd/autism/signs.html

43.   *Stem cell harvest procedure.* (2016). Retrieved from Non Hodgkin Lymphoma
       Cyberfamily: http://www.nhlcyberfamily.org/treatments/collection.htm#-
       methods

44.   *Stem Cell Therapy* . (2016). Retrieved from Stem Cell Institute: https://www.
       cellmedicine.com/stem-cell-therapy-for-osteoarthritis/

45.   *Stem Cell Therapy and spinal cord injury.* (2016). Retrieved from Stem cell
       institute: https://www.cellmedicine.com/stem-cell-therapy-for-spinal-cord-
       injury/

46.   *Stem Cell/Bone Marrow Collection.* (n.d.). Retrieved from Blood and Marrow
       transplant information network: http://www.bmtinfonet.org/before/stem-
       cellmarrowharvest

47.   Terskikh AV, E. M. (2001). From hematopoiesis to neuropoiesis: evidence of
       overlapping genetic programs. *Proc Natl Acad Sci U S A* , 7934-9.

48.   *Tests and Procedures. Hyperbaric Oxygen Therapy.* (1998-2016). Retrieved from
       Mayo Clinic: http://www.mayoclinic.org/tests-procedures/hyperbaric-oxy-
       gen-therapy/basics/why-its-done/prc-20019167

49.   *The Bone Marrow Harvest Procedure.* (1995-2016). Retrieved from Cleveland
       Clinic: http://my.clevelandclinic.org/health/treatments_and_procedures/
       hic_Bone_Marrow_and_Transplantation/hic-bone-marrow-harvest-proce-
       dure

50.   *The Importance of Nutrition before Bone Marrow or Stem Cell Transplant.* (2012).
       Retrieved from Bone Marrow Transplant at Angeles Health International:
       http://www.bonemarrowmx.com/the-importance-of-nutrition-before-bone-
       marrow-transplant-or-stem-cell-transplant/

51.   *Traumatic Brain Injury.* (2016, October 11). Retrieved from Medline Plus:
       https://medlineplus.gov/traumaticbraininjury.html#cat95

52.   *Turning Stem Cells into Insulin-Producing Cells.* (2016). Retrieved from Diabetes
       Research Institute Foundation: https://www.diabetesresearch.org/stem-cells

53.   Weiss, M. L. (2005). Human Umbilical Cord Matrix Stem Cells: Prelimi-
       nary Characterization and Effect of Transplantation in a Rodent Model of
       Parkinson's Disease. *Stem Cells* .

54.   *What are the Causes of TBI?* (2001). Retrieved from Traumatic Brain Injury.
       com: http://www.traumaticbraininjury.com/understanding-tbi/what-are-
       the-causes-of-tbi/

IMMUNOLOGICAL CONDITIONS

RHEUMATOID ARTHRITIS

OVERVIEW:

Rheumatoid arthritis is an autoimmune disease that causes chronic inflammation of the joints. The cells that normally protect our body against foreign invaders mistakenly begin to attack healthy cells. In this case, the cells that line our joints (synovium), cartilage, and bone may also be affected. The resulting inflammation results in reduced mobility and pain in joints.

CAUSE:

Although it is established that this disease has an autoimmune basis, there are other factors that may influence disease development such as:

• Genetics. Research suggests that people who possess

the HLA epitope are 5 times more likely to get rheumatoid arthritis. Some of the genes have been linked to certain genes that are responsible for other autoimmune diseases.

- Environmental Factors. Scientists believe that there may be some triggers in the environment that flare the disease in genetically susceptible individuals. However, there is no known specific cause.

- Hormones. Rheumatoid arthritis has been seen to improve during pregnancy, but flare after it. It is also aggravated during lactation and may worsen with the use of oral contraceptives.

SYMPTOMS:

The symptoms may vary from person to person and depend on which phase the disease is at. The following are some of the hallmark symptoms of rheumatoid arthritis:

- Morning stiffness that lasts more than half an hour

- Joint pain and/or tenderness that has lasted for at least 6 months or longer

- Small joints involvement (wrist, joints of hand and feet)

- Joint involvement is symmetrical

- Along with joints, rheumatoid arthritis can affect other organs of the body when disease activity is high (also known as a 'flare'). [1]

- Dryness, pain, and sensitivity to light in the eyes

- Dryness of mouth or gum infection

- Rheumatoid nodules, which are bony prominences over small joints of the hand or wrist

- Shortness of breath due to scarring in the lungs

- Anemia of chronic disease

HOW STEM CELL THERAPY CAN HELP:

As discussed in previous chapters, pluripotent stem cells taken from the patient's own body pose the least risk in terms of transplant rejection and ethics (as compared to harvesting stem cells from embryos). It is also known that stem cells have the potential to differentiate into new nerves, muscles, and bones.

Mesenchymal stem cells of the bone marrow have been used by researchers in patients with arthritis and these cells not only developed into tissues of mesenchymal origin, but also possess immune regulating mechanisms. T-cell and B-cell activation is suppressed and the use of mesenchymal stem cells in auto-immune diseases has proved to be successful.

In our personal experience we have seen tremendous success with patients with this kind of auto-immune degenerative disease. Specially when using complete bone marrow since is rich with stem cells, rich with stimulant growth factors and rich of other blood components. Our patient's immune system has shown good response in only a few weeks. Regulation and balance acts like a "reset" button on their body, stopping the manifestations of the disorder, stopping further progress and in many cases reversing the side effects caused by such disorder.

PATIENT PREPARATION:

The patient is brought in for thorough evaluation prior to transplantation. The patient meets with a transplant expert who will review his/her medical record, discuss the treatment options and procedures, and will answer any questions that may come with.

If a patient is suffering from pain and inflammation, they will be administered respective medicines to relieve the symptoms before a therapy begins. A proper drug history is also very important as there are certain medicines that must be stopped at least a week before any procedure for example, blood thinners.

It is always a good idea for the body to be replenished continuously by nutrients like vitamins and minerals. Intravenous infusions or special diet may be recommended by a nutritionist or by your family doctor.

STEM CELL SOURCE:

Mesenchymal stem cells are harvested from the patient's bone marrow. As described in chapter 4, usually the patient is given a local anesthetic and aspiration of bone marrow without pain is performed. The target of therapy is immune regulation by suppressing the active proliferation and expression of inflammatory cytokines. This in turn reduces joint inflammation markedly resulting in improved overall symptoms. [2]

STEM CELL PREPARATION:

Complete Bone marrow is preferred to complete this kind of stem cell infusion. There is minimal manipulation and preparation being very careful keeping sterility and high viability of the cells. In some cases additional minerals are added to increase potential of the cells. To ensure negligible damage to the stem cells, no separation process is performed always keeping minimal manipulation of the bone marrow or source of mesenchymal stem cells to the minimum necessary. Fresh bone marrow have shown better engraftment therefore stem cells are not cryopreserved.

STEM CELL INFUSION:

Autologus Stem cells are infused by IV into the blood stream. By not injecting on every joint of the body, big ones and small ones, we avoid poking the patient multiple times and avoid the stress and discomfort of such injections. Stem cells are carried by blood everywhere, which help cover more ground of the immune system.

SECONDARY EFFECTS AND RISKS:

As mentioned above, stem cells are harvested from the patient's own body, hence, there is minimal to no risk of transplant rejection and/or cross contamination. As mentioned in chapter 4, the side effects of a bone marrow aspiration are: Soreness and/or swelling in the following 3 days and maybe a little bleeding on the aspiration site.

There is a positive side effect on this type of infusion and that is because stem cells travel through blood around the body, many of them attach (engraft) to damaged tissue in the internal organs of the body. A regenerative process to those organs takes place, improving their function and efficiency. We have seen an overall wellness benefit with a huge impact to the health of patients.

PSORIATIC ARTHRITIS

OVERVIEW:

Psoriatic arthritis is the chronic inflammation of the skin and joints (inflammatory arthritis). It is usually associated with psoriasis, but its occurrence can be separated from it by years. Psoriasis is a skin condition that causes red, itchy and scaly skin around the elbows, knees, back, buttocks and scalp. While psoriasis is not age-specific, psoriatic arthritis usually affects more adults than the younger age group. [3]

CAUSE:

The underlying pathology of psoriatic arthritis is inflammation (as mentioned above), but research suggests there may be certain factors that trigger his inflammation such as:

• Genes. Research shows that patients with psoriatic arthritis in whom the spine is affected exhibit the gene marker HLA-B27 in about 50% of the cases. Other genes are also involved.

• Immune System. Psoriatic arthritis is linked to auto-immune conditions as well as immunosuppressed conditions such as AIDS in which the number of

T-cells are greatly reduced. This may play a role in the progression of disease in such patients.

- Environmental Factors. The influence of environmental toxins/agents is still undergoing research.

SYMPTOMS:

Psoriasis usually precedes arthritis. The distribution of the signs and symptoms of psoriatic arthritis depends upon the type and the joints involved. Here are some of them: [4]

- Pain in joints. Joints of the fingers, toes, knees, ankle and feet can be involved. There is a pain in the small joints due to inflammation. Sometimes a digit may swell giving it a 'sausage finger' appearance.

- Stiffness. Joint stiffness is usually worse in the mornings. It may mimic RA by having a symmetrical joint involvement.

- Back pain and stiffness in lower back when the sacrum is involved (spondylitis)

- Enthesitis and tendonitis of involved bones.

- Chest pain and shortness of breath may be seen with the involvement of the lung.

HOW STEM CELL THERAPY CAN HELP:

Several clinical studies have shown that stem cell therapy has not only retarded the progression of psoriatic arthritis and psoriasis, but has ameliorated the disease altogether, with a prognosis of a 12-16-year remission phase.

Mesenchymal as well as hematopoietic stem cells have been used for the treatment of this auto-immune disease. Psoriasis with joint inflammation may be associated with other auto-immune diseases as well, such as multiple myeloma as was the case with a middle-aged female with a 20-year history of psoriasis. She presented with a recent history of arthralgia and myalgia. After relevant lab investigations and bone marrow aspiration and biopsy (which showed plasma cells) she was diagnosed with light chain multiple myeloma.

She was treated with high dose steroids as well as a CD 34+ cell transplant. The result was astonishing. She was psoriasis free for 13 years with only mild flares after that which were controlled with anti-inflammatories and the multiple myeloma has remained in remission till date. [5]

PATIENT PREPARATION

The patient is brought in for thorough evaluation prior to transplantation. The patient meets with a transplant expert who will review his/her medical record, discuss the treatment options and procedures, and will answer any questions that may come with.

If a patient is suffering from pain and inflammation, they will be administered respective medicines to relieve the symptoms before beginning therapy. A proper drug history is also very important as there are certain medicines that must be stopped at least a week before any procedure for example, blood thinners.

It is always a good idea for the body to be replenished

continuously by nutrients like vitamins and minerals. Intravenous infusions or special diet may be recommended by a nutritionist or by your family doctor.

STEM CELL SOURCE

Mesenchymal cells can be harvested from a variety of tissues such as bone, adipose tissue and umbilical cord. Hematopoietic stem cells are also extracted from the bone marrow. As described in chapter 4, usually the patient is given a local anesthetic and aspiration of bone marrow without pain is performed. The target of therapy is immune regulation by suppressing the active proliferation and expression of inflammatory cytokines. This in turn reduces chronic inflammation markedly resulting in improved overall symptoms. [2]

STEM CELL PREPARATION

Complete Bone marrow is preferred to complete this kind of stem cell infusion. There is minimal manipulation and preparation being very careful keeping sterility and high viability of the cells. In some cases additional minerals are added to increase potential of the cells. To ensure negligible damage to the stem cells, no separation process is performed always keeping minimal manipulation of the bone marrow or source of mesenchymal stem cells to the minimum necessary. Fresh bone marrow have shown better engraftment therefore stem cells are not cryopreserved.

STEM CELL INFUSION

Intravenous infusion is used for transplant of mesenchymal

cells as well as HSCs. Results are extremely promising with remission of psoriasis and prompt alleviation of arthritis.

By not injecting on every inflammation site of the body, we avoid poking the patient multiple times and avoid the stress and discomfort of such injections. Stem cells are carried by blood everywhere, which help cover more ground of the immune system.

SECONDARY EFFECTS AND RISKS:

There are minimal unwanted side effects. As mentioned above, stem cells are harvested from the patient's own body, hence, there is minimal to no risk of transplant rejection and/or cross contamination. As mentioned in chapter 4, the side effects of a bone marrow aspiration are: Soreness and/or swelling in the following 3 days and maybe a little bleeding on the aspiration site.

There is a positive side effect on this type of infusion and that is because stem cells travel through blood around the body, many of them attach (engraft) to damaged tissue in the internal organs of the body. A regenerative process to those organs takes place, improving their function and efficiency. We have seen an overall wellness benefit with a huge impact to the health of patients.

SYSTEMIC LUPUS

OVERVIEW:

Systemic lupus is a chronic inflammatory condition that involves the immune system. It can affect any part of the body and no two cases are the same. It is common in females of childbearing age; however, studies show that there is a childhood onset of lupus as well. Suspicion should be raised if there is a family history of autoimmune disease.

CAUSE:

Although the exact cause of lupus is unknown, genetics and hormones are thought to play in a role in disease development and progression. Perhaps certain environmental factors are involved as well, but there is no evidence to prove this.

SYMPTOMS:

The signs and symptoms range from mild to severe. Since any part of the body can be affected, there is a wide range of symptoms:

- The most common symptoms are fever, arthralgia and rash.

- Joint pain may be asymmetrical involving the small joints of hands and feet. Common hand deformities include 'swan neck deformity' due to inflammation of the tendons. Avascular necrosis is also common in lupus patients due to high dose steroids taken for treatment. The most common joint affected by AVN is head of femur.

- Skin lesions. There are 3 common cutaneous lesions;

    - Malar/butterfly rash covering the cheeks and bridge of the nose, but sparing the nasolabial folds.

    - Discoid lupus. Round disc shaped lesions/rashes in sun exposed areas with scarring and plaque like. Occurs in about 25% of patients.

    - Photosensitivity. Flares lesions after exposure to the sun that have exacerbated 2 days following sun exposure.

- The kidney is affected in about 50% of patients with systemic lupus, also known as lupus nephritis.

- The lungs may be affected, resulting in pleural effusion, interstitial lung disease, pleuritis etc.

- The most common cardiac lesion is pericarditis. It usually manifests as positional pain that is relieved on leaning forward.

- The gastrointestinal tract is the system which is least affected. However, attention must be paid to secondary bacterial infection of the GIT as lupus is an immune-suppressed state.

HOW STEM CELL THERAPY CAN HELP:

The current conventional treatment for systemic lupus is immunosuppression. This can last for a lifetime and still doesn't provide a cure for the disease. While it does calm down flare ups and mellows disease progression, long term immune suppression can lead to significant morbidity and even mortality.

Hematopoietic stem cell therapy and mesenchymal stem cell therapy have been used for research and clinical trials for the past 15 years and have proved to be promising.

Autologous HSCT has shown to almost cure some patients with severe AD (like lupus) which was not responding to any other treatment.

Mesenchymal cells taken from bone tissue, adipose tissue, skeletal muscle, placenta and other sites functioned as immune-modulators and anti-inflammatory agents. A clinical study showed that MSCs were transplanted in patients with severe SLE and data from a 4 year follow up showed that 50% of the patients entered clinical remission post-transplant. [6]

PATIENT PREPARATION

The patient is brought in for thorough evaluation prior to transplantation. The patient meets with a transplant expert who will review his/her medical record, discuss the treatment options and procedures, and will answer any questions that may come with.

If a patient is suffering from pain and inflammation, they will be administered respective medicines to relieve the symptoms before beginning therapy. A proper drug history is also very

important as there are certain medicines that must be stopped at least a week before any procedure for example, blood thinners.

It is always a good idea for the body to be replenished continuously by nutrients like vitamins and minerals. Intravenous infusions or special diet may be recommended by a nutritionist or by your family doctor.

STEM CELL SOURCE

Mesenchymal cells can be harvested from a variety of tissues such as bone, adipose tissue and umbilical cord. Hematopoietic stem cells are also extracted from the bone marrow. As described in chapter 4, usually the patient is given a local anesthetic and aspiration of bone marrow without pain is performed. The target of therapy is immune regulation by suppressing the active proliferation and expression of inflammatory cytokines. This in turn reduces chronic inflammation markedly resulting in improved overall symptoms. [2]

STEM CELL PREPARATION

Complete Bone marrow is preferred to complete this kind of stem cell infusion. There is minimal manipulation and preparation being very careful keeping sterility and high viability of the cells. In some cases additional minerals are added to increase potential of the cells. To ensure negligible damage to the stem cells, no separation process is performed always keeping minimal manipulation of the bone marrow or source of mesenchymal stem cells to the minimum necessary. Fresh bone marrow have shown better engraftment therefore stem cells are not cryopreserved.

STEM CELL INFUSION

Intravenous infusion is used for transplant of mesenchymal cells as well as HSCs. Patients with lupus tend to be very uncomfortable being touched, injected or any other kind of intervention. By only having one IV we avoid any additional stress and discomfort. Stem cells are carried by blood everywhere, which help cover more ground of the immune system.

SECONDARY EFFECTS AND RISKS:

There are minimal unwanted side effects. As stated above, stem cells are harvested from the patient's own body, hence, there is minimal to no risk of transplant rejection and/or cross contamination. As mentioned in chapter 4, the side effects of a bone marrow aspiration are: Soreness and/or swelling in the following 3 days and maybe a little bleeding on the aspiration site.

There is a positive side effect on this type of infusion and that is because stem cells travel through blood around the body, many of them attach (engraft) to damaged tissue in the internal organs of the body. A regenerative process to those organs takes place, improving their function and efficiency. We have seen an overall wellness benefit with a huge impact to the health of patients.

SJÖGREN'S SYNDROME

OVERVIEW:

Sjögren's syndrome is an autoimmune condition, which is characterized by dryness of the eyes and mouth. The antibodies attack the lacrimation and salivary glands and produce inflammation.

Sjögren's syndrome with isolated dry eyes and mouth, not related to any other autoimmune diseases is called Primary Sjögren's syndrome. When it is related to other connective tissue diseases, such as SLE, it is referred to as Secondary Sjögren's syndrome.

CAUSE:

There may be a genetic predisposition to the disease. It is more common in females around the time of menopause. People with a family history of autoimmune diseases are more prone to get it. Certain environmental factors, like viruses may be involved, although there is no clear proof of this.

SYMPTOMS:

- As mentioned above, dry eyes can lead to irritation and grittiness of the eye, abrasion of the cornea, and inflammation of the eyelids (blepharitis).

- Dry mouth can lead to difficulty in swallowing, dental caries, gum disease, mouth sores, impaired voice, loss of taste, etc.

- Extra-glandular manifestations may include arthralgia, fatigue, Raynaud's phenomenon.

- Associated diseases may be Hashimoto's thyroiditis and biliary cirrhosis

HOW STEM CELL THERAPY CAN HELP:

Stem cell therapy has shown to be effective in the treatment of Sjögren's syndrome. HSCs and MSCs possess innate immune modulating properties, due to which they suppressed autoimmunity, and restored gland function and secretion in Sjögren's syndrome patients. [7]

PATIENT PREPARATION

The patient is brought in for thorough evaluation prior to transplantation. The patient meets with a transplant expert who will review his/her medical record, discuss the treatment options and procedures, and will answer any questions that may come with.

If a patient is suffering from pain and inflammation, they will be administered respective medicines to relieve the symptoms before beginning therapy. A proper drug history is also very important, as there are certain medicines that must be stopped at least a week before any procedure, for example, blood thinners.

It is always a good idea for the body to be replenished continuously by nutrients like vitamins and minerals. Intravenous infusions or special diet may be recommended by a nutritionist or by your family doctor

STEM CELL SOURCE

Mesenchymal cells can be harvested from a variety of tissues such as bone, adipose tissue and umbilical cord. Hematopoietic stem cells are also extracted from the bone marrow. As described in chapter 4, usually the patient is given a local anesthetic and aspiration of bone marrow without pain is performed. The target of therapy is immune regulation by suppressing the active proliferation and expression of inflammatory cytokines. This in turn reduces chronic inflammation markedly resulting in improved overall symptoms. [2]

STEM CELL PREPARATION

Complete Bone marrow is preferred to complete this kind of stem cell infusion. There is minimal manipulation and preparation being very careful keeping sterility and high viability of the cells. In some cases additional minerals are added to increase potential of the cells. To ensure negligible damage to the stem cells, no separation process is performed always keeping minimal manipulation of the bone marrow or source of mesenchymal stem cells to the minimum necessary. Fresh bone marrow have shown better engraftment therefore stem cells are not cryopreserved.

STEM CELL INFUSION

Intravenous infusion is used for transplant of stem cells. Patients with Sjögren's syndrome tend to be very uncomfortable from dryness of the eyes and mouth. By having only one IV we avoid any additional stress and discomfort. Increasing fluids on their system also helps with rehydration. Stem cells are carried by blood everywhere, which help cover more ground of the immune system.

SECONDARY EFFECTS AND RISKS:

There are minimal unwanted side effects. As mentioned above, stem cells are harvested from the patient's own body, hence, there is minimal to no risk of transplant rejection and/or cross contamination. As mentioned in chapter 4, the side effects of a bone marrow aspiration are: Soreness and/or swelling in the following 3 days and maybe a little bleeding on the aspiration site.

There is a positive side effect on this type of infusion and that is because stem cells travel through blood around the body, many of them attach (engraft) to damaged tissue in the internal organs of the body. A regenerative process to those organs takes place, improving their function and efficiency. We have seen an overall wellness benefit with a huge impact to the health of patients.

CROHN'S DISEASE

OVERVIEW:

Crohn's disease is a chronic inflammation of the gut, anywhere from the mouth to the anus. However, more commonly affected part is the end of the small intestine and the beginning of the large intestine. This disease is believed to be an autoimmune condition in which the body's own antibodies react abnormally to the normal gut flora. The exact mechanism is not known. Small ulcers develop in the intestine causing inflammation and erosion.

CAUSE:

As mentioned above, Crohn's disease is an autoimmune condition. It is also believed to have a genetic component, hence, a positive family history is something to look out for. Immune deficiencies and environmental triggers also play a role in disease development in susceptible individuals. Smoking, certain infections, and hormones are risk factors.

SYMPTOMS:

- Abdominal pain

- Diarrhea (may be bloody)

- Weight loss

- Mouth sores

- Blockage of bowel

- Fissures and/or fistulas between organs

HOW STEM CELL THERAPY CAN HELP:

Research suggests that stem cell therapy can help treat Crohn's disease by acting as immune modulators. They are able to repair the damage cells caused by inflammation, by toning down the immune response, inhibiting inflammation, and stimulating tissue repair.

A case study done on a 21-year-old patient with debilitating Crohn's disease underwent HSC therapy for 2 months. On follow up, he showed considerable improvement of symptoms. He had no back pain and abdominal pain, and digestive symptoms had also improved. His stamina and endurance had also improved [10].

Another clinical study was carried out on 45 patients with moderate to severe Crohn's disease, who were resistant to immunosuppressive drugs, not eligible for surgery, and had a morbid quality of life. They were treated with HSCs. On follow up after a year, 9 of them had shown considerable improvement symptomatically as well as endoscopically. [8]

Patients have also shown increase benefits from balancing their immune system and controlling inflammation. It happens that the complete digestive system goes through a regenerative process, therefore the stomach better processes the food ingestion, and intestines have more efficiency on getting nutrients. As a consequence patients state that they feel more energetic, they can eat more diverse food without feeling stomach ache, without reflux, without gut inflammation. The following comment is from an actual patient after two bone marrow autologous stem cell procedures: *"It's really an improvement of the quality of my life in every way. Now I can go to lunch and dinners with friends, I can catch a movie after eating without feeling uncomfortable. I have more energy to exercise, I gained weight, I look healthy."*

PATIENT PREPARATION

The patient is brought in for thorough evaluation prior to transplantation. The patient meets with a transplant expert who will review his/her medical record, discuss the treatment options and procedures, and will answer any questions that may come with.

Since patients are suffering from pain and inflammation, they usually will be taking respective medicines to relieve the symptoms before beginning therapy. A proper drug history is very important as there are certain medicines that must be stopped at least a week before any procedure for example, blood thinners.

It is always a good idea for this kind of patients to be replenished continuously by nutrients like vitamins and minerals. Intravenous infusions or special diet supplements are prescribed. It is recommended to see a nutritionist or a family doctor to monitor blood chemistry, and to guide the patient whenever levels are not balanced.

STEM CELL SOURCE

Mesenchymal cells can be harvested from a variety of tissues such as bone, adipose tissue and umbilical cord. Hematopoietic stem cells are also extracted from the bone marrow. As described in chapter 4, usually the patient is given a local anesthetic and aspiration of bone marrow without pain is performed. The target of therapy is immune regulation by suppressing the active proliferation and expression of inflammatory cytokines. This in turn reduces chronic inflammation markedly resulting in improved overall symptoms. [2]

STEM CELL PREPARATION

Complete Bone marrow is preferred to complete this kind of stem cell infusion. There is minimal manipulation and preparation being very careful keeping sterility and high viability of the cells. In some cases additional minerals are added to increase potential of the cells. To ensure negligible damage to the stem cells, no separation process is performed always keeping minimal manipulation of the bone marrow or source of mesenchymal stem cells to the minimum necessary. Fresh bone marrow has shown better engraftment therefore stem cells are not cryopreserved.

STEM CELL INFUSION

Intravenous infusion is used for transplant of stem cells. Increasing fluids on their system also helps with rehydration. Stem cells are carried by blood everywhere, which help cover more ground of the immune system.

SECONDARY EFFECTS AND RISKS:

Work is continually being done to improve the concerns related to safety of stem cell use. Having said this, autologous stem cell transplant has a lesser chance of graft vs. host rejection, as the cells are taken from the patient's own body.

There are minimal unwanted side effects. As mentioned in chapter 4, the side effects of a bone marrow aspiration are: Soreness and/or swelling in the following 3 days and maybe a little bleeding on the aspiration site.

There is a positive side effect on this type of infusion and that is because stem cells travel through blood around the body, many of them attach (engraft) to damaged tissue in the internal organs of the body. A regenerative process to those organs takes place, improving their function and efficiency. We have seen an overall wellness benefit with a huge impact to the health of patients.

ASTHMA

OVERVIEW:

Asthma is the temporary narrowing of air passages caused by inflammation. Asthma affects about 26 million people in the U.S. and accounts for around 2 million ER visits each year. Asthma can be properly controlled and treated through medicines and inhalers, but it still poses as a dangerous and sometimes even life threatening. It consists of 3 basic stages:

- Airway obstruction

- Airway inflammation

- Airway irritability

CAUSE:

- Infections like sinusitis and flu

- Allergens like pollen, mold, dust etc.

- Smoking

- Exercise (exercise induced asthma)

- Fluctuation in temperature (hot and cold weather)

- Drug induced

SYMPTOMS:

An asthma attack is an acute onset of difficulty in breathing characterized by:

- Coughing

- Wheezing

- Chest tightness

- Shortness of breath

HOW STEM CELL THERAPY CAN HELP:

Stem cell therapy can help delay disease progression and alleviate some of the life threatening symptoms of asthma (and other lung diseases) by regenerating the lung epithelium and restoring glandular function. In addition reducing inflammation factors helped reduce the asthma episodes. Several case studies show that using adult stem cells derived from adipose tissue have proved effective in long-term treatment for asthma.

The results of a recent clinical trial prove that HSCs and MSCs are safe for treating asthma and other lung diseases. The stem cells were derived from the bone marrow and administered to the patients with no infusion related toxicity or adverse effects. At the beginning of the trial, they had elevated levels of C reactive protein (CRP). At a 2-year follow-up, the CRP levels had decreased markedly.[9]

PATIENT PREPARATION

The patient is brought in for thorough evaluation prior to transplantation. The patient meets with a transplant expert who will review his/her medical record, discuss the treatment options and procedures, and will answer any questions that may come with.

If a patient is suffering from pain and inflammation, they will be administered respective medicines to relieve the symptoms before beginning therapy. A proper drug history is also very important as there are certain medicines that must be stopped at least a week before any procedure for example, blood thinners.

STEM CELL SOURCE

Mesenchymal cells can be harvested from a variety of tissues such as bone, adipose tissue and umbilical cord. Hematopoietic stem cells are also extracted from the bone marrow. As described in chapter 4, usually the patient is given a local anesthetic and aspiration of bone marrow without pain is performed.

STEM CELL PREPARATION

Complete Bone marrow is preferred to complete this kind of stem cell infusion. There is minimal manipulation and preparation being very careful keeping sterility and high viability of the cells. In some cases additional minerals are added to increase potential of the cells. To ensure negligible damage to the stem cells, no separation process is performed always keeping minimal manipulation of the bone marrow or source of mesenchymal stem cells to the minimum necessary. Fresh bone marrow has shown better engraftment therefore stem cells are not cryopreserved.

STEM CELL INFUSION

Intravenous infusion is used for transplant of stem cells.

Patients with asthma tend to worsen when they are stressed and agitated. By having only one IV we avoid any additional stress and discomfort. Increasing fluids on their system also helps with rehydration.

SECONDARY EFFECTS AND RISKS:

There are minimal unwanted side effects. As mentioned above, stem cells are harvested from the patient's own body, hence, there is minimal to no risk of transplant rejection and/or cross contamination. As mentioned in chapter 4, the side effects of a bone marrow aspiration are: Soreness and/or swelling in the following 3 days and maybe a little bleeding on the aspiration site.

There is a positive side effect on this type of infusion and that is because stem cells travel through blood around the body, many of them attach (engraft) to damaged tissue in the internal organs of the body. A regenerative process to those organs takes place, improving their function and efficiency. We have seen an overall wellness benefit with a huge impact to the health of patients.

FIBROMYALGIA

OVERVIEW:

This condition refers to chronic pain and tenderness in various 'trigger' areas of the body. Sometimes, even light pressure can cause pain. The pain is described consistent, dull, and aching. If one has experienced this type of pain for at least 3 months, it may favor the diagnosis of fibromyalgia. Some of the common trigger points are:

- Back of the head

- Tips of shoulders

- Upper chest

- Hips

- Knees

- Outer part of elbows

CAUSE:

There is no single certain cause, but several factors are believed to be involved such as:

- Prior infections may trigger fibromyalgia

- Researchers believe that genetic mutations cause fibromyalgia, but genes have not been recognized yet. Family history is important.

- Long-term stress and trauma can lead to hormonal fluctuations which may lead to fibromyalgia

- This condition has been linked with PTSD hence emotional stress and trauma may play a role as well.

SYMPTOMS:

- Pain and tenderness in various trigger points

- Fatigue

- Trouble sleeping

- Depression

- Headaches

- Anxiety

- Dull ache in the lower abdomen

- Difficulty in paying attention

HOW STEM CELL THERAPY CAN HELP:

Several clinical trials have used mesenchymal stem cells to reverse the effects of fibromyalgia. MSCs are transplanted into the patient in multiple stages in the form of CD34+ enriched injections. Controlling the immune system leads to less inflammation and as a consequence less areas of pain. This is a form of targeted regenerative therapy. It promotes healing of damaged tissue.

PATIENT PREPARATION

The patient is brought in for thorough evaluation prior to transplantation. The patient meets with a transplant expert who will review his/her medical record, discuss the treatment options and procedures, and will answer any questions that may come with.

Patient is suffering from pain and inflammation, they are administered respective medicines to relieve the symptoms before beginning therapy. A proper drug history is very important as there are certain medicines that must be stopped at least a week before any procedure for example, blood thinners.

It is always a good idea for the body to be replenished continuously by nutrients like vitamins and minerals. Intravenous infusions may be recommended by a nutritionist or by your family doctor.

A basic psychological evaluation is carried out to see how the patient is dealing with stress and coping strategies. If there is areas of concern, patient is referred to psychological therapy for a deeper evaluation and action plan.

STEM CELL SOURCE

Stem cells are harvested from the patient's bone marrow. As described in chapter 4, usually the patient is given a local anesthetic and aspiration of bone marrow without pain is performed. The target of therapy is immune regulation by suppressing the active proliferation and expression of inflammatory cytokines. This in turn reduces inflammation markedly resulting in improved overall symptoms.

STEM CELL PREPARATION:

Complete Bone marrow is preferred to complete this kind of stem cell infusion. There is minimal manipulation and preparation being very careful keeping sterility and high viability of the cells. In some cases additional minerals are added to increase potential of the cells. To ensure negligible damage to the stem cells, no separation process is performed always keeping minimal manipulation of the bone marrow or source of mesenchymal stem cells to the minimum necessary. Fresh bone marrow have shown better engraftment therefore stem cells are not cryopreserved.

STEM CELL INFUSION:

Autologus Stem cells are infused by only one IV into the blood stream. Avoiding multiple injections avoids the stress and discomfort on the patient. Stem cells are carried by blood everywhere, which helps cover more ground of the immune system.

SECONDARY EFFECTS AND RISKS:

As mentioned above, stem cells are harvested from the patient's own body, hence, there is minimal to no risk of transplant rejection and/or cross contamination. As mentioned in chapter 4, the side effects of a bone marrow aspiration are: Soreness and/or swelling in the following 3 days and maybe a little bleeding on the aspiration site.

There is a positive side effect on this type of infusion and that is because stem cells travel through blood around the body, many of them attach (engraft) to damaged tissue in the internal organs of the body. A regenerative process to those organs takes place, improving their function and efficiency. We have seen an overall wellness benefit with a huge impact to the health of patients.

REFERENCES

1. *Handout on Health: Rheumatoid Arthritis.* (2016, February). Retrieved from National Institute of Arthritis and Musculoskeletal and Skin Diseases: https://www.niams.nih.gov/health_info/rheumatic_disease/#ra_5

2. *ALS Fact Sheet.* (n.d.). Retrieved from National Institute of Neurological Disorders and Stroke: https://www.ninds.nih.gov/Disorders/Patient-Caregiver-Education/Fact-Sheets/Amyotrophic-Lateral-Sclerosis-ALS-Fact-Sheet

3. Augello, A. (2007). Cell therapy using allogeneic bone marrow mesenchymal stem cells prevents tissue damage in collagen-induced arthritis. *Arthritis and Rheumatology* , 1175–1186.

4. Ballabio, F. L. (2009). Stem cell therapy in stroke. *Cellular and Molecular Life Sciences* , 757–772.

5. Behjati, M. (2013). Suggested indications of clinical practice guideline for stem cell-therapy in cardiovascular diseases: A stepwise appropriate use criteria for regeneration therapy. *ARYA Atherosclerosis* , 306-310.

6. *Bone Marrow Aspiration and Biopsy.* (2015). Retrieved from Cancer.Net: http://www.cancer.net/navigating-cancer-care/diagnosing-cancer/tests-and-procedures/bone-marrow-aspiration-and-biopsy

7. Boseley, S. (2015). *First UK patient receives stem cell treatment to cure loss of vision.* London: The Guardian.

8. Centeno, C. (2016, July 18). *8 Ways to increase stem cell health.* Retrieved from Regennex: http://www.regenexx.com/8-ways-improve-your-stem-cells-prior-treatment/

9.   *Chronic liver disease: how could regenerative medicine help?* (2016). Retrieved from Swiss Medica: http://www.startstemcells.com/liver-cirrhosis-treatment.html

10.   Cras, A. (2015). Update on mesenchymal stem cell-based therapy in lupus and scleroderma. *Arthritis Research and Therapy* , 301.

11.   *Diabetes: how could stem cells help?* (2015, November 09). Retrieved from Euro Stem Cell: http://www.eurostemcell.org/factsheet/diabetes-how-could-stem-cells-help

12.   Elvis, A. M. (2011). Ozone therapy: A clinical review. *Journal of Natural Science, Biology and Medicine* , 66–70.

13.   *Exercise triggers stem cells in muscle.* (2012, February 6). Retrieved from Science Daily: https://www.sciencedaily.com/releases/2012/02/120206143944.htm

14.   *Fat Stem Cell Therapy.* (2015). Retrieved from Infinite Horizons Medical Center: http://www.fatstemcelltherapy.com/procedure/

15.   *Handout on Health: Rheumatoid Arthritis.* (2016, February). Retrieved from National Institute of Arthritis and Musculoskeletal and Skin Diseases: https://www.niams.nih.gov/health_info/rheumatic_disease/#ra_5

16.   Helwick, C. (2013, May 22). *Stem Cell Transplantation Halts Crohn's Disease.* Retrieved from Medscape: http://www.medscape.com/viewarticle/804570

17.   Ichim, T. E. (2007). Stem Cell Therapy for Autism. *Journal of Translational Medicine* , 5:30.

18.   Imran Ullah, *. R. (2015). Human mesenchymal stem cells - current trends and future prospective. *Bioscience Reports* , 35 (2).

19.   Jr., W. C. (2017). *Symptoms of psriatic arthritis* . Retrieved from Medicine Net: http://www.medicinenet.com/psoriatic_arthritis/page3.htm

20.   Kehr, W. (2016, October 3). *Ozone Cancer Treatments.* Retrieved from Cancer Tutor: https://www.cancertutor.com/ozone/

21.   Kim, J.-H. (2002). Dopamine neurons derived from embryonic stem cells function in an animal model of Parkinson's disease. *nature, International weekly journal of Science* , 50-56.

22.   Kramerov, A. A. (2015). Stem cell therapies in the treatment of diabetic retinopathy and keratopathy. *Experimental Biology and Medicine* , 559–568.

23.   Iajimi, A. A. (2013). Feasibility of Cell Therapy in Multiple Sclerosis: A Systematic Review of 83 Studies. *International Journal of Hematology-Oncology and Stem Cell Research* , 15-33.

24.   Latham, E. (2016, July 22). *Hyperbaric oxygen therapy.* Retrieved from Medscape: http://emedicine.medscape.com/article/1464149-overview

25.   Lunn, J. S. (2011). Stem Cell Technology for Neurodegenerative Diseases. *Ann Neurology* , 353–361.

26.   Martin R, M. H. (January 24, 2017). Assessment of Patients With Multiple Sclerosis (MS). *National Institute of Neurological Disorders and Stroke (NINDS)* .

27.   Mazzini, L. (2008). Stem cell treatment in Amyotrophic Lateral Sclerosis. *Journal of the Neurological Sciences* , 78–83.

28.   McKhann GM, K. D. (2011). The diagnosis of dementia due to Alzheimer's disease: Recommendations from the National Institute on Aging-Alzheimer's Association workgroups on diagnostic guidelines for Alzheimer's disease. *Alzheimer's and Dementia* , 263-269.

29.   *Motor Neuron Disease Information.* (n.d.). Retrieved from National Institute of Neurological Diseases and Stroke: https://www.ninds.nih.gov/Disorders/All-Disorders/Motor-Neuron-Diseases-Information-Page

30.   Munoz J, S. N. (2014). umbilical cord blood transplantation: past, present, and future. *Stem Cells Transl Med* , 1435-1443.

31.   OM, A.-S. (2011). Stem cell therapy for Alzheimer's disease. *CNS Neurological DIsroders Drug Targets* , 459-85.

32.   Patricia A. Zuk, *. M. (2002). Human Adipose Tissue Is a Source of Multipotent Stem Cells. *Molecular Biology of the Cell* , 4279–4295.

33.   Prof Vincenzo Silani, M. (2004). Stem-cell therapy for amyotrophic lateral sclerosis. *The Lancet* , 200–202.

34.   Richard K. Burt, M., Roumen Balabanov, M., Xiaoqiang Han, M., & al, e. (2015). Association of Nonmyeloablative Hematopoietic Stem Cell Transplantation With Neurological Disability in Patients With Relapsing-Remitting Multiple Sclerosis. *Journal of the American Medical Association (JAMA).* , 275-284.

35.   Riordan, N. (2016). *Stem Cell Therapy* . Retrieved from stem cell Institute: https://www.cellmedicine.com/stem-cell-therapy-for-multiple-sclerosis-3/

36.   Shroff, G. (2016). Human Embryonic Stem Cell Therapy in Crohn's Disease: A Case Report. *The American Journal of Case Reports* , 124–128.

37.   *Signs and Symptoms of ASD*. (n.d.). Retrieved from Centres for Disease Control and Prevention: https://www.cdc.gov/ncbddd/autism/signs.html

38.   *Stem cell harvest procedure*. (2016). Retrieved from Non Hodgkin Lymphoma Cyberfamily: http://www.nhlcyberfamily.org/treatments/collection.htm#-methods

39.   *Stem Cell Therapy* . (2016). Retrieved from Stem Cell Institute: https://www.cellmedicine.com/stem-cell-therapy-for-osteoarthritis/

40.   *Stem Cell Therapy and spinal cord injury*. (2016). Retrieved from Stem cell institute: https://www.cellmedicine.com/stem-cell-therapy-for-spinal-cord-injury/

41.   *Stem Cell/Bone Marrow Collection*. (n.d.). Retrieved from Blood and Marrow transplant information network: http://www.bmtinfonet.org/before/stem-cellmarrowharvest

42.   Sung, S. M. (2015). *Remission of Psoriasis 13 Years After Autologous Stem Cell Transplant*. Parsippany, NJ, USA: Frontline Medical Communications Inc.

43.   Terskikh AV, E. M. (2001). From hematopoiesis to neuropoiesis: evidence of overlapping genetic programs. *Proc Natl Acad Sci U S A* , 7934-9.

44.   *Tests and Procedures. Hyperbaric Oxygen Therapy*. (1998-2016). Retrieved from Mayo Clinic: http://www.mayoclinic.org/tests-procedures/hyperbaric-oxygen-therapy/basics/why-its-done/prc-20019167

45.   *The Bone Marrow Harvest Procedure*. (1995-2016). Retrieved from Cleveland Clinic: http://my.clevelandclinic.org/health/treatments_and_procedures/hic_Bone_Marrow_and_Transplantation/hic-bone-marrow-harvest-procedure

46.   *The Importance of Nutrition before Bone Marrow or Stem Cell Transplant*. (2012). Retrieved from Bone Marrow Transplant at Angeles Health International: http://www.bonemarrowmx.com/the-importance-of-nutrition-before-bone-marrow-transplant-or-stem-cell-transplant/

47.   *Traumatic Brain Injury*. (2016, October 11). Retrieved from Medline Plus: https://medlineplus.gov/traumaticbraininjury.html#cat95

48.   *Turning Stem Cells into Insulin-Producing Cells*. (2016). Retrieved from Diabetes Research Institute Foundation: https://www.diabetesresearch.org/stem-cells

49.   Wang, S. (2010). Non-Invasive Stem Cell Therapy in a Rat Model for Retinal Degeneration and Vascular Pathology. *PLOS one* .

50. Weiss, D. J. (2014). Current Status of Stem Cells and Regenerative Medicine in Lung Biology and Diseases. *Stem Cells* , 16–25.

51. Weiss, J. N. (2015). Stem Cell Ophthalmology Treatment Study (SCOTS) for retinal and optic nerve diseases: a preliminary report. *Neural regeneration research* , 982–988.

52. Weiss, M. L. (2005). Human Umbilical Cord Matrix Stem Cells: Preliminary Characterization and Effect of Transplantation in a Rodent Model of Parkinson's Disease. *Stem Cells* .

53. *What are the Causes of TBI?* (2001). Retrieved from Traumatic Brain Injury. com: http://www.traumaticbraininjury.com/understanding-tbi/what-are-the-causes-of-tbi/

54. *What is Psoriatic arthritis.* (2017). Retrieved from Arhritis Research UK: http://www.arthritisresearchuk.org/arthritis-information/conditions/psoriatic-arthritis/causes.aspx

55. Woods, A. C. (2006). Amelioration of severe psoriasis with psoriatic arthritis for 20 years after allogeneic haematopoietic stem cell transplantation. *Annals of the Rheumatic Diseases* , 65(5): 697.

56. Xu, J. (2012). Allogeneic mesenchymal stem cell treatment alleviates experimental and clinical Sjögren syndrome. *Blood* , 3142–3151.

OPHTHALMOLOGICAL CONDITIONS

RETINITIS PIGMENTOSA

OVERVIEW:

Retinitis pigmentosa is a group of inherited disorders, which causes gradual loss of peripheral vision and night vision disturbances. Degeneration could be relatively fast in a couple of years while other cases could take decades to progress. Eventually, central vision is also compromised.

CAUSE:

This condition is caused by hereditary degeneration of the retina i.e. it is passed on in families. Around 100 genes have been implicated so far.

SYMPTOMS:

- Night vision disturbance is usually the first symptom

- Loss of peripheral vision, also known as tunnel vision

- Loss of central vision

- Problems with color vision may also occur

HOW STEM CELL THERAPY CAN HELP:

Nowadays, there is no treatment for retinitis pigmentosa except gene replacement, that too due to unspecific gene defects. A study was carried out in which pluripotent stem cells were injected into a rat that exhibited retinitis pigmentosa. It was an allogenic transplant, hence, the chances of graft vs. host rejection are less. Stem cell therapy is a method that provides neuro as well as vascular protection. The results were quite impressive. No graft vs. host rejection was seen. While the control specimen had only a single layer of photoreceptors left, the subject had retained 4-5 layers. Visual function had also improved, measured by visual acuity and luminescence threshold. [1]

In humans, there are very few formal studies that could help support a factual experience. There are particular cases treated in Tijuana, Mexico by Dr. Rene Cervantes and Dr. María Eugenia Niño, with formal documented medical files and follow ups for over 12 months, including peripheral view tests and luminescence that show improvements in those particular cases. We are very excited about theses cases, as it could become a major breakthrough in the future.

PATIENT PREPARATION

The patient is brought in for thorough evaluation prior to transplantation. The patient meets with a transplant expert who will review his/her medical record, ophthalmologic tests, discuss the treatment options and procedures, and will answer any questions that may come with.

If a patient is suffering from pain and inflammation, they will be administered respective medicines to relieve the symptoms before beginning therapy. A proper drug history is also very important, as there are certain medicines that must be stopped at least a week before any procedure, e.g. blood thinners.

A simple psychological evaluation is carried out to see how the patient is dealing with stress and coping strategies. It is very uncommon to find psychological issues, since degeneration of sight occurs over a span of considerable time and patient is pretty much adapts to his every day activity with gradually decreasing sight limitations.

STEM CELL SOURCE

Stem cells are usually taken from the patient (autologous) to avoid rejection complications, exsesive inflammation, and any kind of acquired transmittal disease. Stem cells are taken from bone marrow or peripheral blood.

Autologous Hematopoietic cells are usually harvested from bone marrow. As described in chapter 4, usually the patient is given a local anesthetic and aspiration of bone marrow is performed without pain.

Mesenchymal stem cells have also been advocated and

supported through the evidences collected from clinical trials. Therefore, in some cases where the condition of the patient is appropriate, adipose tissue is collected.

STEM CELL PREPARATION

To ensure negligible damage to the stem cells, minimal manipulation of the bone marrow stem cells is necessary. Cells are handled with care. Stem cells are not usually cryopreserved.

Specimen is divided in two parts: One part is usually combined with saline and other cell support reagents. Whereas, the second part is going to be purified and concentrated; the red cells are removed and some plasma is also removed. In this process all captured stem cells inside this components are spinned out into a buffer layer. This layer will be combined with a small volume of plasma obtaining a 1ml to 3 ml concentrated dilution of stem cells.

STEM CELL INFUSION

Part one is infused by IV into the blood stream, expecting to get into the vascularity of the surrounding areas of treatment and maintain the overall wellness of the internal eye of the patient. Whereas, 2nd part of the specimen, the concentrated part as mentioned above, is infused into retrobulbar area of the eye. The goal is to get stem cells near the retina to stimulate all the tissues in the surrounding area too. The retrobulbar injection is given with local anesthesia to eliminate any discomfort.

SECONDARY EFFECTS AND RISKS:

Although there is an extreme quality control while preparing the cells for this kind of injection, there could be some risks involved with the procedure.

The risks are related to contamination and infection. The eye is a very easy area to get contaminated; therefore, sterility of the technique, as well as the facilities and the instruments is of the essence.

The risk involved in a retrobulbar infusion is related to bad positioning of the needle by an inexperienced doctor. A needle puncturing other tissues can produce inflammation, damage, and can even lead to a disability. It is very important that the procedure be performed by a trained and experienced doctor.

Indeed, it is common to get a vein punctured during the procedure and thus is normal to get a black eye the following two days of treatment. This hemorrhage will gradually resolve on its own in around two to three weeks after the procedure.

The side effects of a bone marrow aspiration is soreness and/ or swelling in the following 3 days of the treatment.

Be aware that the retrobulbar injection is not the same as the intrabulbar injection. The intrabulbar route implicates putting the needle inside the eye globe which is riskier and could have severe complications. It is not recommended unless the eye is completely lost, has zero vision, or there is no alternative option.

MACULOPATHY

OVERVIEW:

Maculopathy refers to a damage to the macula (central part of the retina) - the part of the eye that is responsible for central vision. It causes a gradual loss of central vision. Peripheral vision is usually preserved.

CAUSE:

Age related maculopathy

Diabetic maculopathy caused by uncontrolled diabetes. There is usually an accumulation of fluid (edema)

Myopia maculopathy

Exudative maculopathy

Cellophane maculopathy/macular pucker

SYMPTOMS:

Initially the condition is painless, as the normal healthy eye compensates for the affected one. Gradually the symptoms that follow are:

Image metamorphosis. Distortion of the shapes of the images or they may appear smaller than they really are.

When the macula is directly affected, a 'central spot' appears. The patient is unable to see the center of the objects. For instance, he/she/they will be able to see the ears on a head but not the facial expressions on the face.

HOW STEM CELL THERAPY CAN HELP:

Age-related macular degeneration is on the rise and there is no plausible treatment. Injections of anti-endothelial growth factors are being used, but this method is painful and sometimes has to be carried out twice a month.

Stem cell therapy has proved to be a less invasive technique. Recent studies have used pluripotent stem cells, which have the ability to transform into any other cell type. The technique is based on increasing the number of stem cells in the peripheral blood as well as injecting purified concentrated stem cells behind the eye globe by a retrobulbar injection. These stem cells are absorbed by the retrobulbar tissue and regenerate damaged retinal and macular tissue. Vascular regeneration and improved function have also been observed. [3]

A case report of a female patient with age-related macular degeneration was the first UK based person to receive stem cell therapy on experimental basis. The doctors were confident and have been reported to say that they would not have performed it if they didn't think it had potential. Since then, several doctors around the world have repeated this procedure resulting in similar vision improvements. We have seen stem cell therapy has stopped the progression of degenerative maculopathy and in many cases improved night vision as well.

PATIENT PREPARATION

The patient is brought in for thorough evaluation prior to transplantation. The patient meets with a transplant expert who will review his/her medical record, ophthalmologic tests, discuss the treatment options and procedures, and will answer any questions that may come with.

If a patient is suffering from pain and inflammation, they will be administered respective medicines to relieve the symptoms before beginning therapy. A proper drug history is also very important, as there are certain medicines that must be stopped at least a week before any procedure, e.g. blood thinners.

A simple psychological evaluation is carried out to see how the patient is dealing with stress and coping strategies. It is very uncommon to find psychological issues, since degeneration of sight occurs over a span of considerable time and the patient basically adapts to their every day activity with gradually decreasing sight limitations.

STEM CELL SOURCE

Stem cells are usually taken from the patient (autologous) to avoid rejection complications, exsesive inflammation, and any kind of acquired transmittal disease.

Autologous Hematopoietic cells are usually harvested from bone marrow. As described in chapter 4, usually the patient is given a local anesthetic and aspiration of bone marrow is performed without pain.

Mesenchymal stem cells have also been advocated and supported through the evidences collected from clinical trials. Therefore, in some cases where the condition of the patient is appropriate, adipose tissue is collected.

STEM CELL PREPARATION

To ensure negligible damage to the stem cells, minimal manipulation of the bone marrow stem cells is necessary. Cells are handled with care. Stem cells are not usually cryopreserved.

Specimen is divided in two parts: One part is usually combined with saline and other cell support reagents. Whereas, the second part is going to be purified and concentrated; the red cells are removed and some plasma is also removed. In this process all captured stem cells inside this components are spinned out into a buffer layer. This layer will be combined with a small volume of plasma obtaining a 1ml to 3 ml concentrated dilution of stem cells.

STEM CELL INFUSION

Part one is infused by IV into the blood stream, expecting to get into the vascularity of the surrounding areas of treatment and maintain the overall wellness of the internal eye of the patient. Whereas, 2nd part of the specimen, the concentrated part as mentioned above, is infused into retrobulbar area of the eye. The goal is to get stem cells near the retina to stimulate all the tissues in the surrounding area too. The retrobulbar injection is given with local anesthesia to eliminate any discomfort.

SECONDARY EFFECTS AND RISKS:

Although there is an extreme quality control while preparing the cells for this kind of injection, there could be some risks involved with the procedure.

The risks are related tocontamination and infection. The eye is a very easy area to get contaminated; therefore, sterility of the technique as well as the facilities and the instruments is of essence.

The risk involved in a retrobulbar infusion is related to bad positioning of the needle by an inexperienced doctor. A needle puncturing other tissues can produce inflammation, damage, and can lead to other disabilities. Therefore, it is very important that the procedure should be performed by an experienced doctor.

It is common to get a small vein punctured, therefore, it is normal to get a black eye in the following two days of treatment. This hemorrhage will gradually disappear on its own. It may take upto 3 weeks for the whole thing to disappear.

The side effects of a bone marrow aspiration is soreness and/ or swelling in the following 3 days of the treatment.

Beware that the retrobulbar injection is not the same as the intrabulbar injection. The intrabulbar route implicates putting the needle inside the eye globe and that is riskier. It could have severe complications. Thus, it is not recommended unless the eye is completely lost, zero vision, and there is no alternative option.

DIABETIC RETINOPATHY

OVERVIEW:

Diabetic retinopathy refers to a damage to the blood vessels that supply the retina due to increased blood sugar levels in diabetics. This eventually leads to a compromised vision. There are 2 stages of diabetic retinopathy:

Non-proliferative Retinopathy. This is the initial stage and most diabetics have it. Tiny blood vessels swell and begin to leak, and may cause macular edema or become blocked causing macular ischemia. Both of these phenomena lead to a compromised vision.

Proliferative Retinopathy. This is the advanced form of diabetic retinopathy. New vessels begin to form in the retina and sometimes bleed into the vitreous, as they are fragile. Minor bleeding manifests as small floaters in the eye, whereas, major bleeding may cause loss of vision. If these vessels form scar tissue, they can cause retinal detachment.

CAUSE:

As the name indicates, diabetic retinopathy is caused by uncontrolled sugar levels.

SYMPTOMS:

- Blurring of vision, initially

- Floaters in the eye

- Loss of vision

HOW STEM CELL THERAPY CAN HELP:

Stem cell therapy is considered to be the modern era treatment of choice in terms of long term results by targeting the underlying pathogenesis of diabetic retinopathy. Research studies have shown success with stem cell therapy in alleviating underlying abnormalities such as vascular hyperpermeability, capillary closure, and pericyte dropout.

Bone marrow stem cells and mesenchymal stem cells have recently become the preferred choice for retinal regeneration because they can be harvested from multiple sources and expanded in vitro then transplanted intravenously (non-invasive). They also secrete neuroprotective factors, which have proven to be safe in human trials so far. [2]

PATIENT PREPARATION

The patient is brought in for thorough evaluation prior to transplantation. The patient meets with a transplant expert who will review his/her medical record, ophthalmologic tests, discuss the treatment options and procedures, and will answer any questions that may come with.

If a patient is suffering from pain and inflammation, they will be administered respective medicines to relieve the symptoms before beginning therapy. A proper drug history is also very

important, as there are certain medicines that must be stopped at least a week before any procedure, e.g. blood thinners.

A simple psychological evaluation is carried out to see how the patient is dealing with stress and coping strategies. It is very uncommon to find psychological issues, since degeneration of sight occurs over a span of considerable time and patient is pretty much adapts to his every day activity with gradually decreasing sight limitations.

STEM CELL SOURCE

Stem cells are usually taken from the patient (autologous) to avoid rejection complications, exsesive inflammation, and any kind of acquired transmittal disease. Stem cells are taken from bone marrow or peripheral blood.

Autologous Hematopoietic cells are usually harvested from bone marrow. As described in chapter 4, usually the patient is given a local anesthetic and aspiration of bone marrow is performed without pain.

Mesenchymal stem cells have also been advocated and supported through the evidences collected from clinical trials. Therefore, in some cases where the condition of the patient is appropriate, adipose tissue is collected.

STEM CELL PREPARATION

To ensure negligible damage to the stem cells, minimal manipulation of the bone marrow stem cells is necessary. Cells are handled with care. Stem cells are not usually cryopreserved.

Specimen is divided in two parts: One part is usually combined with saline and other cell support reagents. Whereas, the second part is going to be purified and concentrated; the red cells are removed and some plasma is also removed. In this process all captured stem cells inside this components are spinned out into a buffer layer. This layer will be combined with a small volume of plasma obtaining a 1ml to 3 ml concentrated dilution of stem cells.

STEM CELL INFUSION

The first part of the specimen is infused by IV into the blood stream, expecting to get into the vascularity of the surrounding areas of treatment and maintain the overall wellness of the internal eye of the patient. Meanwhile, the second part of the specimen, the concentrated part as mentioned above, is infused into retrobulbar area of the eye. The goal is to get stem cells near the retina to stimulate all the tissues in the surrounding area too. The retrobulbar injection is given with local anesthesia to eliminate any discomfort.

SECONDARY EFFECTS AND RISKS:

Although there is an extreme quality control while preparing the cells for this kind of injection, there could be some risks involved with the procedure.

The risks are related to contamination and infection. The eye is a very easy area to get contaminated; therefore, sterility of the technique as well as the facilities and the instruments is of essence.

The risk involved in a retrobulbar infusion is related to bad positioning of the needle by an inexperienced doctor. A needle puncturing other tissues can produce inflammation, damage, and can lead to other disabilities. Therefore, it is very important that the procedure should be performed by an experienced doctor.

It is common to get a small vein punctured, therefore, it is normal to get a black eye in the following two days of treatment. This hemorrhage will gradually disappear on its own. It may take upto 3 weeks for the whole thing to disappear.

The side effects of a bone marrow aspiration is soreness and/or swelling in the following 3 days of the treatment.

Beware, the retrobulbar injection is not the same as the intrabulbar injection. The intrabulbar route implicates putting the needle inside the eye globe and that is riskier. It could have severe complications. Thus, it is not recommended unless the eye is completely lost, zero vision, and there is no alternative option.

OPTIC NERVE ATROPHY

OVERVIEW:

Optic nerve atrophy is a damage to the optic nerve that leads to loss in central, peripheral, and color vision. The optic nerve carries signals from the eyes to the brain.

CAUSE:

Poor blood flow to the nerve, i.e. ischemic optic neuropathy

Shock

Toxins

Radiation

Trauma

Brain tumors

Multiple sclerosis

Stroke

SYMPTOMS:

Compromised clarity of vision

Compromised field of vision

Ability to see fine details will be lost

Ability of the pupil to react to the light will be lost gradually

HOW STEM CELL THERAPY CAN HELP:

Bone marrow and/or MSCs are ideal to treat optic nerve atrophy because of its multipotent nature. After being injected into the patient, the stem cells begin the process of homing on damaged tissues. Research has shown MSCs to produce photoreceptor like cells in vitro, and transplanted MSCs have shown to exhibit neuroprotective effects in preclinical subjects. There is also substantial evidence supporting HSCs in neurologic and ophthalmic diseases. [4]

PATIENT PREPARATION

The patient is brought in for thorough evaluation prior to transplantation. The patient meets with a transplant expert who will review his/her medical record, ophthalmologic tests, discuss the treatment options and procedures, and will answer any questions that may come with.

If a patient is suffering from pain and inflammation, they will be administered respective medicines to relieve the symptoms before beginning therapy. A proper drug history is also very important, as there are certain medicines that must be stopped at least a week before any procedure, e.g. blood thinners.

A simple psychological evaluation is carried out to see how the patient is dealing with stress and coping strategies. It is very uncommon to find psychological issues, since degeneration of sight occurs over a span of considerable time and patient is pretty much adapts to his every day activity with gradually decreasing sight limitations.

STEM CELL SOURCE

Stem cells are usually taken from the patient (autologous) to avoid rejection complications, exsesive inflammation, and any kind of acquired transmittal disease. Stem cells are taken from bone marrow or peripheral blood.

Autologous Hematopoietic cells are usually harvested from bone marrow. As described in chapter 4, usually the patient is given a local anesthetic and aspiration of bone marrow is performed without pain.

Mesenchymal stem cells have also been advocated and supported through the evidences collected from clinical trials. Therefore, in some cases where the condition of the patient is appropriate, adipose tissue is collected.

STEM CELL PREPARATION

To ensure negligible damage to the stem cells, minimal manipulation of the bone marrow stem cells is necessary. Cells are handled with care. Stem cells are not usually cryopreserved.

Specimen is divided in two parts: One part is usually combined with saline and other cell support reagents. Whereas, the second part is going to be purified and concentrated; the red cells are removed and some plasma is also removed. In this process all captured stem cells inside this components are spinned out into a buffer layer. This layer will be combined with a small volume of plasma obtaining a 1 ml to 3 ml concentrated dilution of stem cells.

STEM CELL INFUSION

Part one is infused by IV into the blood stream, expecting to get into the vascularity of the surrounding areas of treatment and maintain the overall wellness of the internal eye of the patient. Whereas, 2nd part of the specimen, the concentrated part as mentioned above, is infused into retrobulbar area of the eye. The goal is to get stem cells near the retina to stimulate all the tissues in the surrounding area too. The retrobulbar injection is given with local anesthesia to eliminate any discomfort.

SECONDARY EFFECTS AND RISKS:

Although there is an extreme quality control while preparing the cells for this kind of injection, there could be some risks involved with the procedure.

The risks are related tocontamination and infection. The eye is a very easy area to get contaminated; therefore, sterility of the technique as well as the facilities and the instruments is of essence.

The risk involved in a retrobulbar infusion is related to bad positioning of the needle by an inexperienced doctor. A needle puncturing other tissues can produce inflammation, damage, and can lead to other disabilities. Therefore, it is very important that the procedure should be performed by an experienced doctor.

It is common to get a small vein punctured, therefore, it is normal to get a black eye in the following two days of treatment.

This hemorrhage will gradually disappear on its own. It may take upto 3 weeks for the whole thing to disappear.

The side effects of a bone marrow aspiration is soreness and/or swelling in the following 3 days of the treatment.

Beware, the retrobulbar injection is not the same as the intrabulbar injection. The intrabulbar route implicates putting the needle inside the eye globe and that is riskier It could have severe complications. Thus, it is not recommended unless the eye is completely lost, zero vision, and there is no alternative option.

REFERENCES

1.   Wang, S. (2010). Non-Invasive Stem Cell Therapy in a Rat Model for Retinal Degeneration and Vascular Pathology. *PLOS one*.

2.   Kramerov, A. A. (2015). Stem cell therapies in the treatment of diabetic retinopathy and keratopathy. *Experimental Biology and Medicine*, 559–568.

3.   *ALS Fact Sheet*. (n.d.). Retrieved from National Institute of Neurological Disorders and Stroke: https://www.ninds.nih.gov/Disorders/Patient-Caregiver-Education/Fact-Sheets/Amyotrophic-Lateral-Sclerosis-ALS-Fact-Sheet

4.   Ballabio, F. L. (2009). Stem cell therapy in stroke. *Cellular and Molecular Life Sciences* , 757–772.

5.   Behjati, M. (2013). Suggested indications of clinical practice guideline for stem cell-therapy in cardiovascular diseases: A stepwise appropriate use criteria for regeneration therapy. *ARYA Atherosclerosis* , 306-310.

6.   *Bone Marrow Aspiration and Biopsy*. (2015). Retrieved from Cancer.Net: http://www.cancer.net/navigating-cancer-care/diagnosing-cancer/tests-and-procedures/bone-marrow-aspiration-and-biopsy

7.   Boseley, S. (2015). *First UK patient receives stem cell treatment to cure loss of vision.* London: The Guardian.

8. Centeno, C. (2016, July 18). *8 Ways to increase stem cell health*. Retrieved from Regennex: http://www.regenexx.com/8-ways-improve-your-stem-cells-prior-treatment/

9. *Chronic liver disease: how could regenerative medicine help?* (2016). Retrieved from Swiss Medica: http://www.startstemcells.com/liver-cirrhosis-treatment.html

10. *Diabetes: how could stem cells help?* (2015, November 09). Retrieved from Euro Stem Cell: http://www.eurostemcell.org/factsheet/diabetes-how-could-stem-cells-help

11. Elvis, A. M. (2011). Ozone therapy: A clinical review. *Journal of Natural Science, Biology and Medicine* , 66–70.

12. *Exercise triggers stem cells in muscle.* (2012, February 6). Retrieved from Science Daily: https://www.sciencedaily.com/releases/2012/02/120206143944.htm

13. *Fat Stem Cell Therapy*. (2015). Retrieved from Infinite Horizons Medical Center: http://www.fatstemcelltherapy.com/procedure/

14. Ichim, T. E. (2007). Stem Cell Therapy for Autism. *Journal of Translational Medicine* , 5:30.

15. Imran Ullah, *. R. (2015). Human mesenchymal stem cells - current trends and future prospective. *Bioscience Reports* , 35 (2).

16. Kehr, W. (2016, October 3). *Ozone Cancer Treatments*. Retrieved from Cancer Tutor: https://www.cancertutor.com/ozone/

17. Kim, J.-H. (2002). Dopamine neurons derived from embryonic stem cells function in an animal model of Parkinson's disease. *nature, International weekly journal of Science* , 50-56.

18. Kramerov, A. A. (2015). Stem cell therapies in the treatment of diabetic retinopathy and keratopathy. *Experimental Biology and Medicine* , 559–568.

19. lajimi, A. A. (2013). Feasibility of Cell Therapy in Multiple Sclerosis: A Systematic Review of 83 Studies. *International Journal of Hematology-Oncology and Stem Cell Research* , 15-33.

20. Latham, E. (2016, July 22). *Hyperbaric oxygen therapy*. Retrieved from Medscape: http://emedicine.medscape.com/article/1464149-overview

21. Lunn, J. S. (2011). Stem Cell Technology for Neurodegenerative Diseases. *Ann Neurology* , 353–361.

22. Martin R, M. H. (January 24, 2017). Assessment of Patients With Multiple Sclerosis (MS). *National Institute of Neurological Disorders and Stroke (NINDS)* .

23. Mazzini, L. (2008). Stem cell treatment in Amyotrophic Lateral Sclerosis. *Journal of the Neurological Sciences* , 78–83.

24. McKhann GM, K. D. (2011). The diagnosis of dementia due to Alzheimer's disease: Recommendations from the National Institute on Aging-Alzheimer's Association workgroups on diagnostic guidelines for Alzheimer's disease. *Alzheimer's and Dementia* , 263-269.

25. *Motor Neuron Disease Information.* (n.d.). Retrieved from National Institute of Neurological Diseases and Stroke: https://www.ninds.nih.gov/Disorders/ All-Disorders/Motor-Neuron-Diseases-Information-Page

26. Munoz J, S. N. (2014). umbilical cord blood transplantation: past, present, and future. *Stem Cells Transl Med* , 1435-1443.

27. OM, A.-S. (2011). Stem cell therapy for Alzheimer's disease. *CNS Neurological DIsroders Drug Targets* , 459-85.

28. Patricia A. Zuk, *. M. (2002). Human Adipose Tissue Is a Source of Multipotent Stem Cells. *Molecular Biology of the Cell* , 4279–4295.

29. Prof Vincenzo Silani, M. (2004). Stem-cell therapy for amyotrophic lateral sclerosis. *The Lancet* , 200–202.

30. Richard K. Burt, M., Roumen Balabanov, M., Xiaoqiang Han, M., & al, e. (2015). Association of Nonmyeloablative Hematopoietic Stem Cell Transplantation With Neurological Disability in Patients With Relapsing-Remitting Multiple Sclerosis. *Journal of the American Medical Association (JAMA).* , 275-284.

31. Riordan, N. (2016). *Stem Cell Therapy* . Retrieved from stem cell Institute: https://www.cellmedicine.com/stem-cell-therapy-for-multiple-sclerosis-3/

32. *Signs and Symptoms of ASD.* (n.d.). Retrieved from Centres for Disease Control and Prevention: https://www.cdc.gov/ncbddd/autism/signs.html

33. *Stem cell harvest procedure.* (2016). Retrieved from Non Hodgkin Lymphoma Cyberfamily: http://www.nhlcyberfamily.org/treatments/collection.htm#-methods

34. *Stem Cell Therapy* . (2016). Retrieved from Stem Cell Institute: https://www. cellmedicine.com/stem-cell-therapy-for-osteoarthritis/

35. *Stem Cell Therapy and spinal cord injury*. (2016). Retrieved from Stem cell institute: https://www.cellmedicine.com/stem-cell-therapy-for-spinal-cord-injury/

36. *Stem Cell/Bone Marrow Collection*. (n.d.). Retrieved from Blood and Marrow transplant information network: http://www.bmtinfonet.org/before/stem-cellmarrowharvest

37. Terskikh AV, E. M. (2001). From hematopoiesis to neuropoiesis: evidence of overlapping genetic programs. *Proc Natl Acad Sci U S A* , 7934-9.

38. *Tests and Procedures. Hyperbaric Oxygen Therapy*. (1998-2016). Retrieved from Mayo Clinic: http://www.mayoclinic.org/tests-procedures/hyperbaric-oxygen-therapy/basics/why-its-done/prc-20019167

39. *The Bone Marrow Harvest Procedure*. (1995-2016). Retrieved from Cleveland Clinic: http://my.clevelandclinic.org/health/treatments_and_procedures/hic_Bone_Marrow_and_Transplantation/hic-bone-marrow-harvest-procedure

40. *The Importance of Nutrition before Bone Marrow or Stem Cell Transplant*. (2012). Retrieved from Bone Marrow Transplant at Angeles Health International: http://www.bonemarrowmx.com/the-importance-of-nutrition-before-bone-marrow-transplant-or-stem-cell-transplant/

41. *Traumatic Brain Injury*. (2016, October 11). Retrieved from Medline Plus: https://medlineplus.gov/traumaticbraininjury.html#cat95

42. *Turning Stem Cells into Insulin-Producing Cells*. (2016). Retrieved from Diabetes Research Institute Foundation: https://www.diabetesresearch.org/stem-cells

43. Wang, S. (2010). Non-Invasive Stem Cell Therapy in a Rat Model for Retinal Degeneration and Vascular Pathology. *PLOS one* .

44. Weiss, J. N. (2015). Stem Cell Ophthalmology Treatment Study (SCOTS) for retinal and optic nerve diseases: a preliminary report. *Neural regeneration research* , 982–988.

45. Weiss, M. L. (2005). Human Umbilical Cord Matrix Stem Cells: Preliminary Characterization and Effect of Transplantation in a Rodent Model of Parkinson's Disease. *Stem Cells* .

46. *What are the Causes of TBI?* (2001). Retrieved from Traumatic Brain Injury. com: http://www.traumaticbraininjury.com/understanding-tbi/what-are-the-causes-of-tbi/

ORTHOPEDIC CONDITIONS

KNEE ARTHROSIS

OVERVIEW:

Arthrosis of the knee joint is a degenerative condition, in which the cartilage covering the opposing ends of the joint disintegrates due to chronic and constant wear and tear. Arthrosis can affect any joint in the body. Arthrosis leads to increased friction between the articulating bones of the joint. The patient may not feel the effects of arthrosis for a long time.

Arthrosis comprises of an inactive or painless phase known as 'silent arthrosis' and a painful phase known as 'active arthrosis'. As the cartilage degenerates, it also affects the bone surfaces resulting in the formation of osteophytes (bony projections).

CAUSE:

- Age related

- Obesity

- Trauma injury

- Infections

- Inflammation

- Occupational arthrosis

SYMPTOMS:

- Pain in knee (or any other affected joint)

- Stiffness related to movement

- Pain after periods of inactivity

- Morning pain is common until joints 'warm up'

- Swollen knee or increased tendency of swelling of joints

- Decreased motion/flexibility of joints

HOW STEM CELL THERAPY CAN HELP:

The current treatment of arthrosis or arthritis, i.e. physiotherapy and drugs only provides temporary relief. To recover the cartilage structure and function has remained a challenge mainly because is a tissue without nutrition of vessels, once damages autoregeneration becomes really hard. Severe cases are treated with total knee replacement surgery, which are extremely expensive and may not always yield long-lasting results. Usually a knee replacement lasts 10-15 yrs depending on the habits of the patient. Therefore a very active young person could go through several knee replacements on his life.

It is common to push back to the future a surgery as long as the patient can, to limit one knee/hip replacement in his life, but sometimes living that time with pain is a cost not so convenient.

Recent research suggests that stem cell therapy can help restore a normal cartilage and bone function. Mesenchymal stem cells are preferred as they are multipotent, found in several tissues, including the fluid inside the joints and are able to maintain their multipotency in vitro and in vivo. They produce chondrogenic cells. [1]

Bone Marrow stem cells infused with its natural growth factors and stimulants gives nutrition to the cartilage to promote its regeneration.

PATIENT PREPARATION

The patient is brought in for thorough evaluation prior to transplantation. The patient meets with a transplant expert who will review his/her medical record, X-rays, discuss the treatment options and procedures, and will answer any questions that may come with.

If a patient is suffering from pain and inflammation, they will be administered respective medicines to relieve the symptoms before beginning therapy. A proper drug history is also very important as there are certain medicines that must be stopped at least a week before any procedure for example, blood thinners.

It is always a good idea for the body to be replenished continuously by nutrients like vitamins and minerals.

Intravenous infusions may be recommended by a nutritionist.

A psychological evaluation is carried out to see how the patient is dealing with stress and coping strategies.

STEM CELL SOURCE

Bone marrow stem cells or adipose tissue stem cells work very well in cartilage regeneration. MSCs are processed from adipose tissue while bone marrow is taken from a big bone in the body such as iliac crest or tibia bone.

STEM CELL PREPARATION

Complete Bone marrow is sometimes the best bet to complete this kind of stem cell infusion. In these cases there is not much preparation more than being very careful keeping sterility and other safety measures. Since adipose tissue stem cells work very good as well, fat tissue is mini-lipoaspirated from the belly of the patient and then MSCs are separated by centrifugation and other purification steps. The aim is to increase the cartilage build-up. The chondrogenic activity of the harvested cells is evaluated, as well as glycosaminoglycan and type II collagen deposition, before reinjection.

STEM CELL INFUSION

Stem cells are injected directly into the joint (intra-articular). Experience of the doctor is really significant on this step to avoid injecting on tissues not related but nearby, as well as to achieve that the stem cells stay to the area of care and not to "travel" out of the damaged zone. When in doubt ultrasound machines could be useful to guide the doctor of such injection.

SECONDARY EFFECTS AND RISKS:

MSC therapy has a significant advantage to traditional surgical approaches such as autologous chondrocyte transplantation: cartilage biopsy is not needed, thus no external stress and cellular damage are applied at the donor-site articular surface. Moreover, direct intra-articular injection of the MSC is a simpler way to treat advanced osteoarthritis of the knee.

Patients could expect some inflammation of the knee for 24-48 hrs, with some pain related to inflammation. Usually analgesic is facilitated for the first 24 hrs. Load to the knee (such as exercise or long walks) is not recommended for a few days.

REPAIR OF SPINAL-CORD INJURIES

OVERVIEW:

Spinal cord injury is a disconnection or loss of nerve tissue due to an insult to the spinal cord and nerves, resulting in loss of sensory, motor, or autonomic function. Such patients often have disabilities and neurological impairment.

CAUSE:

- Leading cause is motor vehicle accidents

- Falls make the elderly more vulnerable to SCI

- Personal assaults like gunshot wounds

- Tumors

- Vascular disorders

- Infections

- Spondylosis

- Iatrogenic injuries (after epidural, spinal tap, etc.)

- Osteoporosis

SYMPTOMS:

The symptoms of spinal cord injury depend upon the spinal cord segment that is injured and the severity of injury. Lower injury segments will affect lower extremities while upper segments will affect functions of th upper body. Incomplete injuries will affect function while a complete spinal cord injury will imply a complete loss of function.

- Loss of complete or some sensation

- Loss of complete or some motor function

- Loss of bladder and bowel control

- Altered sexual function, sensitivity, and fertility

- Intense pain or increased sensitivity to pain

- Difficulty breathing or coughing

HOW STEM CELL THERAPY CAN HELP:

Current conventional treatments for spinal cord injury are largely supportive and palliative, but do not restore normal function of damaged nerves. However, pluripotent stem cells can at some level. They can be infused with the intention to differentiate into neural tissue and then replace the damaged cells in spinal cord injury or help the regeneration of stimulants for nerves to reconnect.

Research suggests that adult stem cells have the potential to not only produce new neurons, but also exhibit neuro-protective properties leading to anatomical as well as functional recovery. Studies on myelin deficient mice have shown that stem cells were able to form oligodendriocytes and myelinated axons after transplant. Human MSCs show a great promise. [2]

Proper expectation must be understood by the patients in any case, but most importantly on these cases. In our experience we have seen benefits such as improving sensation, some bladder and bowel control but very little on motor function, an overall increase of organ function and better blood tests. We find it very unethical to give false expectations to the patient and to overpromise the potential of stem cells. Living with spinal cord injury is a very difficult situation and in the practical day-to-day activities the change we find after stem cell therapy is very little.

PATIENT PREPARATION

The patient is brought in for thorough evaluation prior to transplantation. The patient meets with a transplant expert who will review his/her medical record, discuss the treatment options and procedures, and will answer any questions that may come with.

If a patient is suffering from pain and inflammation, they will be administered respective medicines to relieve the symptoms before beginning therapy. A proper drug history is also very important as there are certain medicines that must be stopped at least a week before any procedure for example, blood thinners.

It is always a good idea for the body to be replenished continuously by nutrients like vitamins and minerals. Intravenous infusions or special diet may be recommended by a nutritionist or by your family doctor.

A simple psychological evaluation is carried out to see how

the patient is dealing with stress and coping strategies. If there are psychological concerns a deeper evaluation is ordered.

STEM CELL SOURCE

Autologous Hematopoietic cells are used to treat this condition. Usually harvested from bone marrow. As described in chapter 4, usually the patient is given a local anesthetic and aspiration of bone marrow without pain is performed.

Mesenchymal stem cells have also been advocated and supported through the evidence collected from clinical trials. Therefore in some cases where the condition of the patient is appropriate adipose tissue is collected .

We have heard of a few places where Embryonic stem cells have been used to treat this condition, but ethical issues still remain. HSCs or MSCs are found in several sources and can be extracted easily, hence, making it the preferred choice.

STEM CELL PREPARATION

To ensure negligible damage to the stem cells, minimal manipulation of the bone marrow stem cells is necessary. Cells are handled with care. Stem cells are not usually cryopreserved.

A specimen is divided in two parts: One part is usually combined with saline and other cell support reagents. While the second part is going to be concentrated; the red cells are removed, and some plasma is also removed. In this process all captured stem cells inside this components are spinned out into a buffer layer. This layer will be combined with a small volume of plasma obtaining a 1 ml - 3 ml concentrated dilution of stem cells.

STEM CELL INFUSION

Part one is infused by IV into the blood stream, they will help the overall wellness of the internal organs of the body. And part 2, the concentrated part mentioned above, is infused into the spinal cord and at the level of injury. The goal is to get stem cells near the injury to stimulate all the tissues in the surrounding area too. The spinal injection is performed with local anesthesia to eliminate any discomfort.

SECONDARY EFFECTS AND RISKS:

The side effects of a bone marrow aspiration are soreness and/or swelling in the following 3 days.

For the spinal infusion there could be signs of soreness and redness. The risk involved in an spinal infusion is related to a bad positioning of the needle by and inexperienced doctor.

A needle puncturing other tissues can produce inflammation, damage to nerves that can lead to other disabilities

Another risk to be aware of is contamination and infection. The zone of the spinal cord injury has little to no immunologic system, therefore very easy to get contaminated and damaged.

OSTEOARTHRITIS

OVERVIEW:

Osteoarthritis is a degenerative disease of the joints. In fact, it is the most common condition that affects around 27 million Americans. More commonly involved joints are the knees, hips, lower back and neck, small joints of the fingers, and the bases of the thumb and big toe.

Osteoarthritis occurs when the protective cartilaginous tissue covering the opposing surfaces of the bone begins to disintegrate, causing the rubbing of bones against each other during movement. This results in inflammation, pain, and tenderness, and limits the movement of the joint. Bits of bone may chip off and float around in the joint, worsening the ongoing process of inflammation.

CAUSE:

- Age. The most common cause.

- Genes. There may be a genetic component to the development of osteoarthritis. For instance, there is a condition in which the collagen forming gene is absent. This causes osteoarthritis in people as young as 20 years.

- Obesity. Being overweight increases the stress on the weight bearing joints, and increases the wear and tear process.

- Injury and overuse. Ligament and tendon injuries and fractures can lead to osteoarthritis. Certain professions that require standing for long periods of time and weight lifting can also increase the chances of osteoarthritis.

SYMPTOMS:

- Stiffness in the morning or after a period of inactivity

- Pain

- Limited movement

- Crackling of the joints on bending

- Mild swelling around the joint

- Difficulties in performing daily tasks may also occur

HOW STEM CELL THERAPY CAN HELP:

Stem cell therapy has provided the potential to reverse the degenerative process of osteoarthritis. Current treatment aims to relieve the pain and inflammation through drugs. Physiotherapy aims to improve movement, but cannot reverse the damage that has already been done.

Clinical trials have shown evidence of Stem cell therapy to improve the overall symptoms of patients suffering with mild to moderate osteoarthritis. MSCs are chosen as they are multi-potent, accessible, least immunogenic, possess immuno-suppressive properties, and are easy to grow in culture. [3]

PATIENT PREPARATION

The patient is brought in for thorough evaluation prior to transplantation. The patient meets with a transplant expert who will review his/her medical record, X-rays, discuss the treatment options and procedures, and will answer any questions that may come with.

If a patient is suffering from pain and inflammation, they will be administered respective medicines to relieve the symptoms before beginning therapy. A proper drug history is also very important as there are certain medicines that must be stopped at least a week before any procedure for example, blood thinners.

It is always a good idea for the body to be replenished continuously by nutrients like vitamins and minerals. Intravenous infusions or special diet may be recommended by a nutritionist or by your family doctor.

A simple psychological evaluation is carried out to see how the patient is dealing with stress and coping strategies. If there are psychological concerns a deeper evaluation is ordered.

STEM CELL SOURCE

Bone marrow stem cells or adipose tissue stem cells work very well in cartilage regeneration. MSCs are processed from adipose tissue while bone marrow is taken from a big bone in the body such as iliac crest or tibia bone.

STEM CELL PREPARATION

Complete Bone marrow is sometimes preferd to complete this kind of stem cell infusion. In these cases there is not much preparation more than being very careful keeping sterility and other safety measures. Since adipose tissue stem cells work very good as well, fat tissue is mini-lipoaspirated from the belly of the patient and then MSCs are separated by centrifugation and other purification steps. The aim is to increase the cartilage build-up. The chondrogenic activity of the harvested cells is evaluated, as well as glycosaminoglycan and type II collagen deposition, before reinjection.

STEM CELL INFUSION

Stem cells are injected directly into bigger joints (intra-articular). Smaller joints are rarely treated since will implicate many mini injections with too much discomfort. An additional Intravenous Stem cell solution is recommended to balance the immune factor and help with the natural healing of the smaller joints.

SECONDARY EFFECTS AND RISKS:

MSC therapy has a significant advantage to traditional surgical approaches such as autologous chondrocyte transplantation: cartilage biopsy is not needed, thus no external stress and cellular damage are applied at the donor-site articular surface. Moreover, direct intra-articular injection of the MSC is a simpler way to treat advanced osteoarthritis.

Patient could expect some inflammation of the joints being treated for 24-48 hrs, with some pain related to inflammation.

Usually analgesic is facilitated for the first 24 hrs. Exercise is not recommended for a few days.

The side effects of a bone marrow aspiration is soreness and/or swelling in the following 3 days.

REFERENCES

1.   Uth, K. (2014). Stem cell application for osteoarthritis in the knee joint: A minireview. World Journal of Stem cells , 629–636.

2.   Tewarie, R. S. (2009). Stem Cell–Based Therapies for Spinal Cord Injury. The Journal of Spinal Cord Medicine, 105–114.

3.   DAVATCHI, F. (2011). Mesenchymal stem cell therapy for knee osteoarthritis. Preliminary report of four patients. International Journal of Rheumatic Diseases, 211–215.

METABOLIC CONDITIONS

DIABETES MELLITUS

OVERVIEW:

Diabetes mellitus is a group of metabolic diseases characterized by high blood sugar (glucose) levels that result from defects in insulin secretion, or its action, or both. Diabetes mellitus, commonly referred to as diabetes was first identified as a disease associated with "sweet urine," and excessive muscle loss in the ancient world. Elevated levels of blood glucose (hyperglycemia) lead to spillage of glucose into the urine, hence the term sweet urine.

Normally, blood glucose levels are tightly controlled by insulin, a hormone produced by the pancreas. Insulin lowers the blood glucose level. When the blood glucose elevates, insulin is released from the pancreas to normalize the glucose level by promoting the uptake of glucose into body cells. In patients with diabetes, the absence of insufficient production of or an inability of the body to properly use insulin causes hyperglycemia. Diabetes is a chronic medical condition, meaning that although it can be controlled, it lasts a lifetime.

Diabetes is one of the top 10 leading causes of morbidity and mortality, affecting nearly 350 million people worldwide. [1] Diabetes mellitus is a devastating and complex metabolic disease, associated with severe long-term micro- and macro-vascular complications, and carries a high rate of morbidity and mortality when patients do not pay the attention to it. A number of medical risks are associated with Diabetes. Many of them stem from damage to the tiny blood vessels in your eyes (called diabetic retinopathy), nerves (diabetic neuropathy), and kidneys (diabetic nephropathy).

CAUSE:

Diabetes causes vary depending on your genetic makeup, family history, ethnicity, health and environmental factors. There is no common diabetes cause that fits every type of diabetes.

The two types of diabetes are referred to as type 1 and type 2.

Type 1 diabetes, also called insulin-dependent diabetes. It used to be called juvenile-onset diabetes, because it often begins in childhood. Is caused by the immune system destroying the cells in the pancreas that make insulin. This causes diabetes by leaving the body without enough insulin to function normally. This is called an autoimmune reaction, or autoimmune cause, because the body is attacking itself. Genetic disposition may be the stronger cause for Diabetes Type 1.

There are no specific diabetes causes, but the following triggers may be involved: Viral or bacterial infection, Chemical toxins within food, unidentified component causing autoimmune reaction

Diabetes type 2 was also called non-insulin-dependent or adult-onset diabetes; By far, is the most common form of diabetes accounting for 95% of diabetes cases in adults, but with the epidemic of obese and overweight kids, more teenagers are now developing type 2 diabetes. It results from an inadequate mass of insulin-producing pancreatic beta cells, characterized by a relative deficiency of β-Cell, impaired β-cell function with insulin resistance in peripheral organs[1].

Type 2 diabetes causes are usually multifactorial - more than one diabetes cause is involved. Often, the most overwhelming factor is a family history of type 2 diabetes. There are a variety of risk factors, any or all of which increase the chances of developing the condition. These include: Obesity, Living a sedentary lifestyle, Increasing age, Bad diet, sometimes pregnancy or illness can trigger the cascade of metabolic environment leading to diabetes type 2.

There are a variety of other potential diabetes causes. These include the following:

Pancreatitis is known to increase the risk of developing diabetes, as is a pancreatectomy.

Polycystic Ovary Syndrome (PCOS). One of the root causes of PCOS is obesity-linked insulin resistance, which may also increase the risk of pre-diabetes and type 2 diabetes.

Cushing's syndrome. This syndrome increases production of the cortisol hormone, which serves to increased blood glucose levels. An over-abundance of cortisol can cause diabetes.

Glucagonoma. Patients with glucagonoma may experience diabetes because of a lack of equilibrium between levels of insulin production and glucagon production.

Steroid induced diabetes (steroid diabetes) is a rare form of diabetes that occurs due to prolonged use of glucocorticoid therapy.

SYMPTOMS:

People who think they might have diabetes must visit a physician for diagnosis. They might have some or none of the following symptoms:

- Frequent urination

- Excessive thirst

- Unexplained weight loss

- Extreme hunger

- Sudden changes in vision

- Tingling or numbness in hands or feet

- Feeling very tired most of the time

- Very dry skin

- Sores that are slow to heal

- More infections than usual

HOW STEM CELL THERAPY CAN HELP:

Pluripotent cells taken from the patient's own body poses the least risk in terms of transplant rejection. Mesenchymal stem cells of the bone marrow have been used by researchers in patients with both types of Diabetes and these cells not only stimulating insulin production but also the adequate use of it in the body. Several factors have been found to promote proliferation of β-cells. It has been demonstrated that β-cells have the ability to sustain themselves through slow replication. However, the mechanism remains unclear and the numbers of new β-cells are inadequate. Almost twenty years ago, pancreatic duct cells were found to possess the ability to form new islets with β-like cells. Therefore, pancreatic duct epithelial cells are assumed to represent the main source of stem cells for pancreatic regeneration.

In our personal experience we have seen significant success with patients with type 1 Diabetes. Specially when using complete bone marrow that possess immune regulating mechanisms since is rich of stem cells, rich of stimulant growth factors and rich of other blood components.

Our patient's have shown good response in only a few weeks. You cannot expect to stop insulin consumption but lowering the dose and frequency are common. A regulation and balance process begins, stopping further progress of degeneration and preventing the long term effects caused by diabetes. Of course, this is not magic, all patients, specially type 2, have to continue with periodic exercise routine and good eating habits.

PATIENT PREPARATION

The patient is brought in for thorough evaluation prior to transplantation. The patient meets with a transplant expert who will review his/her medical record, discuss the treatment options and procedures, and will answer any questions that may come with.

A couple of weeks before procedure, the patient must commit to a healthy lifestyle (eating habits and exercise). These habits will help get most out of stem cell therapy and starts the chain of beneficial effects of diabetes control. If this commitment is not in place, patient will feel better only for a few weeks after procedure and in the long run will be at the same point where he/she/they started.

If a patient is suffering from pain and inflammation, they will be administered respective medicines to relieve the symptoms before a therapy begins. A proper drug history is also very important as there are certain medicines that must be stopped at least a week before any procedure for example, blood thinners.

STEM CELL SOURCE

Stem cells are usually taken from the patient (autologous) bone marrow to avoid rejection complications, excessive inflammation, and any kind of acquired transmittal disease.

Autologous Hematopoietic cells are usually harvested from bone marrow. As described in chapter 4, usually the patient is given a local anesthetic and aspiration of bone marrow is performed without pain.

Mesenchymal stem cells have also been advocated and supported through the evidences collected from clinical trials.

Therefore, in some cases where the condition of the patient is appropriate, adipose tissue is collected. Mesenchymal stem cells (MSCs) have a pro-angiogenic and immunomodulatory properties and the remarkable ability to expand, making them extremely attractive from a therapeutic perspective.

STEM CELL PREPARATION

Complete Bone marrow is preferred to complete this kind of stem cell infusion. There is minimal manipulation and preparation being very careful keeping sterility and high viability of the cells. In some cases additional minerals are added to activate potential of the cells. To ensure negligible damage to the stem cells, no separation process is performed always keeping minimal manipulation of the bone marrow or source of mesenchymal stem cells to the minimum necessary. Fresh bone marrow have shown better engraftment therefore stem cells are not cryopreserved.

STEM CELL INFUSION

The solution is infused by IV into the blood stream, Stem cells travel into the vascular system of the body to maintain overall wellness of the patient's organs and trigger autoimmune balance. Many stem cells get into the pancreatic tissue regenerating islets with β-like cells.

There is the possibility of using concentrated stem cells to infuse into the pancreas directly, but we find this method to be more risky, invasive, expensive, with a slower patient recovery and the outcome is slightly higher than only IV. It is worthwhile repeating an IV infusion a few months later compared to a direct injection to the pancreas.

SECONDARY EFFECTS AND RISKS:

Stem cells are harvested from the patient's own body, hence, there is minimal to no risk of transplant rejection and/or cross contamination. As mentioned in chapter 4, the side effects of a bone marrow aspiration are: Soreness and/or swelling in the following 3 days and maybe a little bleeding on the aspiration site.

There are positives side effects on this type of infusion. Because stem cells travel through blood around the body, many of them attach (engraft) to damaged tissue in the internal organs of the body. Stem cells get all the way to tiny veins and arteries helping with vascularization, therefore improving areas such as vision, kidney, numbness of extremities, etc. A regenerative process to those organs takes place, improving their function and efficiency. We have seen an overall wellness benefit with a huge impact to the health of patients.

HEART INSUFFICIENCIES AND CARDIOMYOPATHY

OVERVIEW:

Having heart insufficiency means that for some reason your heart is not pumping blood around the body as well as it should be. Therefore there is the inability of the heart to keep up with the demands and fails to pump blood with normal efficiency. When this occurs, an inadequate blood flow gets to vital organs such as the brain, liver and kidneys Cardiomyopathy is a disease of the heart muscle, sometimes acquire, sometimes hereditary disease of the heart muscles that make it hard for the heart to deliver blood to the body and can lead to heart failure [3].

CAUSE:

There are lots of reasons why someone might be diagnosed with heart problems. It can be sudden or it can happen slowly over months or even years. Etiology is multifactorial, including genetic and/or environmental causes. The genetic etiology is known in less than 20% of the cases.

The most common causes are: heart attack, high blood pressure, cardiomyopathy (hereditary or caused by other viral infections) [3].

It can also be caused by: heart valve problems, alcohol or recreational drugs, vitamin deficiency, an uncontrolled irregular heart rhythm (arrhythmia), congenital heart conditions (ones you're born with), and some cancer treatments.

SYMPTOMS:

Symptoms occur because the heart does not have enough strength to pump blood all the way round the body efficiently. This can cause fluid to pool in the feet and legs. If this fluid is left unmanaged, it can build and spread to your stomach area and sit beneath your lungs. This reduces their ability to expand and makes you short of breath.

Therefore the most common symptoms are:

- Breathlessness

- Swollen legs and feet

- Chest pain

- Dizziness

- Fatigue

- Loss of appetite

- Weight gain

HOW STEM CELL THERAPY CAN HELP:

Regenerative medicine is known as looking at new ways to repair heart muscle that's been damaged as a result of a heart attack in people with heart failure. It includes looking at how stem cells can become heart muscle cells to help with this repair. Recent studies have shown that cardiac stem cells have similar features as bone marrow cells. These cells are clonogenic and have the ability to differentiate themselves from cardiomyocytes, vascular smooth muscle cells, and endothelial cells. Human pluripotent stem cells, provide a renewable resource of cells that can be differentiated into virtually any somatic cell type in the body. The technology provides a renewable source of functional cardiomyocytes[4]. The aim of therapy is to improve the pumping function of the heart.

Stem cells have been used in tissue engineering of all three cardiac valves. While the bone marrow mesenchymal stem cells (BM-MSCs) can certainly be used for tissue engineering through manipulation, by themselves they can engraft and regenerate damaged tissue as long as have not become scar. BM-MSCs maintain a selective advantage in terms of genetic stability and immunosuppression [4].

Identification of cardiac stem cells (CSC) in the adult heart activated by acute myocardial infarctions (AMI) supported the argument. AMI demands myocardial repair, causing resident CSC to re-enter the cell cycle and circulating stem cells to move to the injury site. Early studies suggested that non-cardiac stem cells transdifferentiate into cardiomyocytes and repair damaged myocardium.

PATIENT PREPARATION

The patient is brought in for thorough evaluation prior to transplantation. The patient meets with a transplant expert who will review his/her medical record, discuss the treatment options and procedures, and will answer any questions that may come with.

If a patient is suffering from pain and inflammation, they will be administered respective medicines to relieve the symptoms before beginning therapy. A proper drug history is also very important, as there are certain medicines that must be stopped at least a week before any procedure, e.g. blood thinners.

It is always a good idea for the body to be replenished continuously by nutrients like vitamins and minerals. Intravenous infusions or special diet may be recommended by a nutritionist or by your family doctor.

STEM CELL SOURCE

From the standpoint of cardiac tissue specificity, cardiovascular progenitor cells taken from vascular structures have been extensively used for valve engineering. Stem cells are usually taken from the patient (autologous) bone marrow to avoid rejection complications, excessive inflammation, and any kind of acquired transmittal disease.

Autologous stem cells are harvested from the patient's bone marrow. As described in chapter 4, usually the patient is given a local anesthetic and aspiration of bone marrow without pain is performed.

STEM CELL PREPARATION

A variety of stem cells derived from different sources have been used in tissue-engineered pulmonary valves. The ideal stem cell must maintain extensive differentiation and proliferative capacity, which has been demonstrated in BM-MSCs. The prototypical cell source must also be well characterized; it has to be easily accessible and easy to culture to obtain clinically relevant numbers. BM-MSCs are particularly advantageous in this regard.

BM SC goes through minimal manipulation and preparation being very careful keeping sterility and high viability of the cells. In some cases additional minerals are added to activate potential of the cells. To ensure negligible damage to the stem cells, no separation process is performed always keeping minimal manipulation of the bone marrow. Fresh bone marrow have shown better engraftment therefore stem cells are not cryopreserved.

STEM CELL INFUSION

Peripheral intravenous infusion is an indirect method with favourable outcomes. It is simple and non-invasive, relying on post-AMI physiological signals to target cells towards damaged tissues.

Direct intramyocardial injection during coronary artery bypass graft (CABG) surgery easily allows stem cells to be placed into the targeted zone. Transendocardial injection is similar to the intramyocardial route, but uses a flexible catheter-based percutaneous technique across the aortic valve. Injecting cells in and around the infarct zone allow greater cell engraftment, while using fewer cells. Intracoronary infusion into the infarct-related artery is the most popular in AMI trials. The cells are injected via catheter into the affected artery. We find this method to be more risky, invasive, expensive, with a slower patient recovery; since the outcome is slightly higher than only IV, we rather repeat an IV infusion a few months later compared to a direct injection to the myocardium.

SECONDARY EFFECTS AND RISKS:

Direct intramyocardial injection has the risks of an standard coronary artery bypass and possible thromboembolic events following transplantation. Potential risks include myocardial perforation, AMI, and induction of ventricular arrhythmias [5]. Therefore we preferred IV infusion where there are minimal secondary effects.

Stem cells are harvested from the patient's own body, hence, there is minimal to no risk of transplant rejection and/or cross contamination. As mentioned in chapter 4, the side effects of a bone marrow aspiration are: Soreness and/or swelling in the following 3 days and maybe a little bleeding on the aspiration site.

HEPATIC INSUFFICIENCY

OVERVIEW:

The liver is a vital organ (the second largest organ in the body), it is responsible for processing everything you eat and drink. It converts food and drinks into energy and nutrients for your body to use. It produces proteins important for the blood and clotting, it filters out harmful substances, toxins, metabolizes drugs and alcohol, removes them from our blood, and helps our body fight off infections.

Liver, or hepatic, disease refers to conditions that may harm the liver and decrease its ability to function normally. Liver disease, whether acute or chronic, can pose a significant risk to one's health. Many factors can contribute to the risk of developing chronic liver disease: lifestyle behaviours, genetics, and medications.

In those with liver damage, the liver may eventually stop functioning correctly. Liver failure is an extremely serious condition, and you should receive treatment immediately even a liver transplant may be needed in some cases. Liver failure and liver diseases are major health problems worldwide, leading to high mortality and also one of the high health care costs. Millions of patients die due to liver pathologies and diseases every year throughout the world.

Liver insufficiency can occur suddenly or gradually. Many people do not have any liver damage symptoms until serious liver problems have already developed slowly and silently. Chronic liver failure indicates that the liver has been failing gradually, possibly for years. It can take months or even years before you exhibit any symptoms.

One of the easiest ways to prevent liver failure is to moderate drinking levels. For healthy women and men over age of 65 it is recommended to limit alcohol consumption to one drink per day while in healthy men under 65 should consume no more than two drinks per day.

CAUSE:

Chronic liver failure occurs if the liver has lost most or all of its function. This condition can be caused by hepatitis infection, reaction to medications, alcohol abuse, advance fatty liver, etc.

One of the most common causes is the result of cirrhosis, which is usually caused by long-term alcohol usage. Cirrhosis occurs when healthy liver tissue is replaced with scar tissue.

Exposure to harmful chemicals or viruses harm this organ too, different liver diseases such as:

• Hepatitis B & C

• Alcohol-related Liver Disease

• Non-alcoholic Fatty Liver Disease (NAFLD) & Non-alcoholic Steatohepatitis (NASH)

• Autoimmune Hepatitis

- Bile duct disease such as Primary Biliary Cirrhosis (PBC) and Primary Sclerosing Cholangitis (PSC)

- Metabolic diseases such as Hemochromatosis, Wilson disease and Alpha-1 antitrypsin deficiency

SYMPTOMS:

One of the most common chronic liver disease symptoms is jaundice, yellowing of your skin and eyes. Other symptoms may include:

- Pain areas in the abdomen

- Fatigue

- Nausea

- Yellow skin and eyes

- Water electrolyte imbalance

- Diarrhea

- Bruising or bleeding easily

- Edema, or fluid buildup in the legs

- Ascites, or fluid buildup in the abdomen

- Hair loss

- Itchy skin

- Dark urine or tar-colored stool

- Weakness or muscle loss

- Loss of appetite and weight loss

- Curling of fingers

- Spider-like veins

These symptoms can also be attributed to other problems or disorders, which can make liver failure hard to diagnose. Some people don't have any signs until their liver failure has progressed to an advanced stage. An advance stage shows toxins build up in the brain and cause sleeplessness, mental disorientation and confusion, lack of concentration, and even decreased mental function. This patient may also experience an enlarged spleen, stomach bleeding, and kidney failure.

HOW STEM CELL THERAPY CAN HELP:

Medication for liver disease depends on which liver condition a patient has. For many conditions, medications do not serve as a "cure," but rather as long-term treatment so that the liver disease is controlled and complications from chronic liver disease do not develop.

When liver insufficiency is diagnosed on early stages, stem cells can be a good idea to improve efficiency of the organ. MSCs have proven to have a high potential for liver regeneration. Stem cells engraft and differentiate into hepatocyte-like cells with the ability to colonize the liver after injury and function similarly to mature hepatocytes.

Stem cells combined with proper diet modifications could stabilize the condition and prevent future complications and a liver transplant. Since your liver plays a crucial role in digestion and works to removes toxins, diet and nutrition are critical in maximizing its ability to function properly. Avoid alcohol, high sodium, sugar, and saturated fats from your diet, and replace them with cruciferous and green leafy vegetables, healthy fats, and lean protein.

If the diagnosis becomes liver failure, meaning there is too much scar tissue (cirrhosis) and very low function of the organ; stem cells have a hard time repairing the damaged tissue. Most likely the patient will get recommendation of an organ transplant. Even though stem cells work very little on liver repair at this point, there are other benefits that should be taken on consideration. Circulatory stem cells help the rest of the organs staying in a better shape and as a consequence the complete body of the patient becomes a stronger recipient of the organ transplant. In addition, they offer another advantage: they have immunomodulatory or immunosuppressive properties that down-regulate T cell, B cell, and NK cell function. Clinically, this can translate into the ability to induce a better tolerance after liver transplantation.

PATIENT PREPARATION

The patient is brought in for thorough evaluation prior to transplantation. The patient meets with a transplant expert who will review his/her medical record, discuss the treatment options and procedures, and will answer any questions that may come with.

If a patient is suffering from pain and inflammation, they will be administered respective medicines to relieve the symptoms before beginning therapy. A proper drug history is also very important, as there are certain medicines that must be stopped at least a week before any procedure, e.g. blood thinners.

It is always a good idea for the body to be replenished continuously by nutrients like vitamins and minerals. Intravenous infusions or special diet may be recommended by a nutritionist or by your family doctor.

STEM CELL SOURCE

Stem cells can be obtained from either Adipose or Bone marrow. Bone marrow-derived stem cells include hematopoietic and mesenchymal stem cells (MSCs). Autologous stem cells are harvested from the patient's bone marrow. As described in chapter 4, usually the patient is given a local anesthetic and aspiration of bone marrow without pain is performed.

STEM CELL PREPARATION

Complete bone marrow is preferred to complete this kind of stem cell infusion. There is minimal manipulation and preparation being very careful keeping sterility and high viability of the cells. In some cases additional minerals are added to increase potential of the cells. To ensure negligible damage to the stem cells, no separation process is performed always keeping minimal manipulation of the bone marrow or source of mesenchymal stem cells to the minimum necessary. Fresh bone marrow have shown better engraftment therefore stem cells are not cryopreserved.

STEM CELL INFUSION

Intravenous infusion is used for transplant of mesenchymal cells as well as HSCs.   By only having one IV we avoid any additional stress and discomfort to the patient. Stem cells are carried by blood everywhere, and being the liver the second largest organ in the body, it will filter the stem cells from the blood and take those tools to start the regenerative process. Since blood carry stem cells everywhere this method helps cover other areas of the body getting other organs spare stem cells for an overall wellness.

SECONDARY EFFECTS AND RISKS:

There are minimal unwanted side effects.   As above, stem cells are harvested from the patient's own body, hence, there is minimal to no risk of transplant rejection and/or cross contamination. As mentioned in chapter 4, the side effects of a bone marrow aspiration are: Soreness and/or swelling in the following 3 days and maybe a little bleeding on the aspiration site.

RENAL INSUFFICIENCY

OVERVIEW:

The kidneys are very important organs in body function, not only by filtering the blood and getting rid of waste products, but also by balancing the electrolyte levels in the body, and stimulating the production of red blood cells. Normally, the kidneys regulate body fluid and blood pressure, as well as regulate blood chemistry.

When blood flows to the kidney, sensors within specialized kidney cells regulate how much water to excrete as urine, along with what concentration of electrolytes. This system is controlled by renin, a hormone produced in the kidney that is part of the fluid and blood pressure regulation systems of the body[8]. Kidneys are also the source of erythropoietin in the body, a hormone that stimulates the bone marrow to make red blood cells. Special cells in the kidney monitor the oxygen concentration in blood. If oxygen levels fall, erythropoietin levels rise and the body starts to manufacture more red blood cells.   Kidneys together with the liver are the organs that filter waste products from the blood.

Renal insufficiency is poor function of the kidneys that may be due to a reduction in blood-flow to the kidneys caused by renal artery disease. Proper kidney function may be disrupted, however, when the arteries that provide the kidneys with blood become narrowed, a condition called renal artery stenosis. Some patients with renal insufficiency experience no symptoms or only mild symptoms. Others develop dangerously high blood pressure, poor kidney function, or kidney failure that requires dialysis.

Chronic renal failure results in the accumulation of fluid and waste products in the body, causing low urine output and waste accumulation. These may occur without symptoms. Most bodily systems are affected by chronic renal failure.

Since most people have two kidneys, both kidneys must be damaged for complete kidney failure to occur. Fortunately, if only one kidney fails or is diseased it can be removed, and the remaining kidney may continue to have normal kidney (renal) function. If both patient's kidneys are injured or diseased, a donor kidney(s) may transplanted.

CAUSE:

The causes of renal insufficiency are diverse, ranging from genetic factors, family history, old age, hyperlipidemia, hypertension to smoking, renal artery diseases, glomerulonephritis of any type (one of the most common causes), polycystic kidney disease, hypertension, Alport syndrome, reflux nephropathy, obstruction, kidney stones, infection, and analgesic toxicity. Diabetes mellitus is a major cause of chronic renal failure [8]. Kidney failure may occur from an acute situation that injures the kidneys or from chronic diseases that gradually cause the kidneys to stop functioning.

SYMPTOMS:

Initially kidney failure may cause no symptoms (asymptomatic). As kidney function decreases, the symptoms are related to the inability to regulate water and electrolyte balances, clear waste products from the body, and promote red blood cell production. Build-up of waste products and excess fluid in the body may cause weakness, shortness of breath, lethargy, swelling, and confusion. Inability to remove potassium from the bloodstream may lead to abnormal heart rhythms and in some cases sudden death.

If the following symptoms of kidney insufficiency are not controlled they could complicate the case developing into life-threatening circumstances.

- Decrease urine production

- Generalized edema

- Problems concentrating

- Fatigue

- Nausea, vomiting

- Shortness of breath

- Generalized weakness due to anemia

- Loss of appetite

- Congestive heart failure

- Metabolic acidosis

- High blood potassium (hyperkalemia)

- Heart rhythm disturbances (arrhythmias)

- Rising urea levels in the blood (uremia)

- Protein-energy malnutrition

- Loss of lean body mass

HOW STEM CELL THERAPY CAN HELP:

The purpose of Stem cell therapy in renal insufficiency is to avoid complications of renal disease such as anemia, heart disease, malnutrition, and bone disease. These all develop long before the onset of renal failure. Even though stem cells are not considered a cure, they could help a patient on stopping or slowing the degenerative process. It is obvious that going through a kidney transplant has implied risks and side effects, keeping your own kidney with some function is preferred than a transplant.

In recent years, it has been shown that functional stem cells exist in the adult bone marrow, and they can contribute to renal remodelling or reconstitution of injured renal glomeruli, especially mesangial cells, and hMSC found in renal glomeruli differentiated into mesangial cells in vivo after glomerular injury occurred.

Mesenchymal stem cells form a population of self-renewing, multipotent cells that can be isolated from several tissues. Multiple preclinical studies have demonstrated that the administration of exogenous MSC could prevent renal injury and could promote renal recovery through a series of complex mechanisms, in particular via immunomodulation of the immune system and release of paracrine factors and microvesicles.

There are patients who do not have a choice and need a kidney transplant right away. Unfortunately there is no source of human parts available at any given moment and compatibility between donor and recipient adds another factor to the formula. After being added to the "waiting list" for a compatible organ, there is valuable time not to be wasted. Since it can take months for your organ to become available, patients are highly recommended to stay as healthy as they can. The success rate of a kidney transplant increases substantially when the recipient has an overall good health. Stem cells, nutrition and physical activity (supervised by your caregiver) can help maintaining the patient healthier than just waiting passively.

PATIENT PREPARATION

The patient is brought in for thorough evaluation prior to transplantation. The patient meets with a transplant expert who will review his/her medical record, discuss the treatment options and procedures, and will answer any questions that may come with.

If a patient is suffering from pain and inflammation, they will be administered respective medicines to relieve the symptoms before beginning therapy. A proper drug history is also very important, as there are certain medicines that must be stopped at least a week before any procedure, e.g. blood thinners.

It is always a good idea for the body to be replenished continuously by nutrients like vitamins and minerals. Intravenous infusions or special diet may be recommended by a nutritionist or by your family doctor.

STEM CELL SOURCE

Stem cells can be obtained from either Adipose or Bone marrow. Bone marrow-derived stem cells include hematopoietic and mesenchymal stem cells (MSCs). Autologous stem cells are harvested from the patient's bone marrow. As described in chapter 4, usually the patient is given a local anesthetic and aspiration of bone marrow without pain is performed. Kidney stem cells have been isolated from other organs. It has been shown that functional stem cells exist in the adult bone marrow.

STEM CELL PREPARATION

Complete Bone marrow is preferred to complete this kind of stem cell infusion. There is minimal manipulation and preparation being very careful keeping sterility and high viability of the cells. In some cases additional minerals are added to increase potential of the cells. To ensure negligible damage to the stem cells, no separation process is performed always keeping minimal manipulation of the bone marrow or source of mesenchymal stem cells to the minimum necessary. Fresh bone marrow have shown better engraftment therefore stem cells are not cryopreserved.

STEM CELL INFUSION

Intravenous infusion is used for transplant of mesenchymal cells as well as HSCs. By only having one IV we avoid any additional stress and discomfort to the patient as well as control the fluid amount being introduced to the body. Stem cells are carried by blood everywhere, and being natural filters of the body, they will extract the stem cells from the blood and take those tools to start the regenerative process. Since blood carry stem cells everywhere this method helps cover other areas of the body getting other organs spare stem cells for an overall wellness.

SECONDARY EFFECTS AND RISKS:

There are minimal unwanted side effects. As it is mentioned above, stem cells are harvested from the patient's own body, hence, there is minimal to no risk of transplant rejection and/or cross contamination. As mentioned in chapter 4, the side effects of a bone marrow aspiration are: Soreness and/or swelling in the following 3 days and maybe a little bleeding on the aspiration site.

CHRONIC OBSTRUCTIVE PULMONARY DISEASE

OVERVIEW:

Chronic obstructive pulmonary disease (COPD) is a group of progressive lung diseases. The disease gets progressively worse over time if not treated early. Most people who have COPD have one or two related lung illnesses. These most common illnesses are chronic bronchitis and emphysema.

Chronic bronchitis is when the airways in the lungs become red, inflammation and narrowing of the bronchial tubes are present, allowing hypersecretion of thick and stretchy mucus to build up. The mucus makes it hard to breathe. Sometimes it is accompanied by a chronic productive cough (more than 4 months).

Emphysema slowly destroys the alveolar walls distal to the terminal bronchiole, without significant pulmonary fibrosis, which interferes with outward airflow, limiting getting oxygen into the blood and carbon dioxide out of it. That's what makes it more difficult to exhale (breathe out).

CAUSE:

COPD is caused by damage to the lungs. It's a disease that takes a long time to develop. Damage occurs from breathing in unhealthy substances constantly and over time. This includes air pollution, chemical fumes, gases, vapors, or mists, tobacco smoke (including second-hand smoke), and dust.

The top cause of COPD is smoking followed by long-term exposure to chemical irritants. Most people with COPD are over 40 years old and have at least some history of smoking. The longer you smoke, the greater your risk of COPD is. About 90 percent of people who have COPD are smokers or former smokers.

Some risk factors of developing COPD are asthma, workplaces where forced to be exposed to chemicals and fumes, as well as inhaling dust activities. Also often poorly ventilated homes, forcing families to breathe fumes from cooking and heating fuel.

There may be a genetic predisposition to developing COPD. Up to 5 percent of people with COPD have a deficiency in a protein called alpha-1-antitrypsin. This deficiency causes the lungs to deteriorate and also can affect the liver.

SYMPTOMS:

COPD makes it harder to breathe. Symptoms may be quite mild at first, you might even dismiss them as a cold, beginning with coughing and shortness of breath. As it progresses, it can become increasingly difficult to breathe.

Early symptoms include:

• Occasional shortness of breath, especially

after exercise

- Mild but recurrent cough

As the lungs become more damaged, you may experience:

- Shortness of breath, after even mild exercise such as walking up a flight of stairs

- Wheezing, or noisy breathing

- Chest tightness

- Chronic cough, with or without mucus

- Need to clear mucus from your lungs every day

Frequent and long lasting cough, colds, flu, or other respiratory infections

- Fatigue

- Hypoxic spells

- Dizziness

HOW STEM CELL THERAPY CAN HELP:

Chronic obstructive pulmonary disease (COPD) is chronic and irreversible airway inflammation. Currently, there is no curative treatment for COPD. Delaying treatment can lead to complications, such as heart problems (irregular heartbeat and heart failure), high blood pressure, and respiratory infections. Infections that can further damage the lungs.

The main goals of COPD management are to mitigate symptoms and improve patients' quality of life. Stem cell-based therapy offers a promising therapeutic approach that has shown potential in diverse degenerative lung diseases.

Mesenchymal stem cells (MSCs) are known to give rise to several cell types, including osteoblasts, chondrocytes, adipocytes, stroma cells, and skeletal myoblasts; they can differentiate into endothelial cell types. In clinical studies, MSC treatment has shown promising results in diverse lung disorders, including emphysema, bronchopulmonary dysplasia, fibrosis, and acute respiratory distress syndrome. MSCs has been shown to reduce tissue degeneration, through secretion of paracrine factors such as epidermal growth factor.

Stem cells have been proposed to interfere with inflammatory responses and exert immunomodulatory effects. MSCs have been found to show profound suppressive effects on immune cells and pathways and recent researches have demonstrated that MSCs suppress lung injury, inflammation and immune-mediated lung diseases. Moreover, MSCs have antifibrotic activity and hold great therapeutic potential for treating pulmonary fibrosis. The most widely studied cell types are bone marrow-derived MSCs (BM-MSCs) and adipose-derived MSCs (AD-MSCs)

PATIENT PREPARATION

The patient is brought in for thorough evaluation prior to transplantation. The patient meets with a transplant expert who will review his/her medical record, discuss the treatment options and procedures, and will answer any questions that may come with.

If a patient is suffering from pain and inflammation, they will be administered respective medicines to relieve the symptoms before beginning therapy. A proper drug history is also very

important, as there are certain medicines that must be stopped at least a week before any procedure, (e.g. blood thinners).

It is always a good idea for the body to be replenished continuously by nutrients like vitamins and minerals. Intravenous infusions or special diet may be recommended by a nutritionist or by your family doctor.

STEM CELL SOURCE

The ideal stem cell need not only be pluripotent, but must maintain extensive differentiation and proliferative capacity. Stem cells obtained from either Adipose or Bone marrow have this characteristics. Bone marrow-derived stem cells include hematopoietic and mesenchymal stem cells (MSCs). Autologous stem cells are harvested from the patient's bone marrow. As described in chapter 4, usually the patient is given a local anesthetic and aspiration of bone marrow without pain is performed.

STEM CELL PREPARATION

Complete Bone marrow is preferred to complete this kind of stem cell infusion. There is minimal manipulation and preparation being very careful keeping sterility and high viability of the cells. In some cases additional minerals are added to increase potential of the cells. To ensure negligible damage to the stem cells, no separation process is performed always keeping minimal manipulation of the bone marrow or source of mesenchymal stem cells to the minimum necessary[11]. Fresh bone marrow has shown better engraftment therefore stem cells are not cryopreserved.

STEM CELL INFUSION

In regards to cell-based therapy in lung diseases, systemic delivery is usually through vascular route, such as intravenous (IV) infusion. Intravenous infusion is used for transplant of mesenchymal cells as well as HSCs. By having one IV we avoid any additional stress and discomfort to the patient. No direct injection into the organ is need it. Stem cells are carried by blood everywhere, and lungs being one of the first organ to be after blood pumping by the heart; the stem cells engraft to different parts of the lung helping the regenerative process. Since blood carry stem cells everywhere in the body, this method helps cover other organs for an overall wellness.

SECONDARY EFFECTS AND RISKS:

There are minimal unwanted side effects.

As mentioned above, stem cells are harvested from the patient's own body, hence, there is minimal to no risk of transplant rejection and/or cross contamination. As mentioned in chapter 4, the side effects of a bone marrow aspiration are: Soreness and/or swelling in the following 3 days and maybe a little bleeding on the aspiration site.

REFERENCES

1. Young HE, Duplaa C, Katz R, Thompson T, Hawkins KC, Boev AN, Henson NL, Heaton M, Sood R, Ashley D, Stout C, Morgan JH, 3rd, Uchakin PN, Rimando M, Long GF, Thomas C, Yoon JI, Park JE, Hunt DJ, Walsh NM, Davis JC, Lightner JE, Hutchings AM, Murphy ML, Boswell E, McAbee JA, Gray BM, Piskurich J, Blake L, Collins JA, Moreau C, Hixson D, Bowyer FP, 3rd, Black AC., Jr Adult-derived stem cells and their potential for use in tissue repair and molecular medicine. J Cell Mol Med. 2005;9:753–769. [PubMed]

2. Mai ML, Ahsan N, Gonwa T. 2006. The long-term management of pancreas transplantation. Transplantation 82(8):991-1003.

3. J. M. Hare, J. E. Fishman, G. Gerstenblith et al., "Comparison of allogeneic vs autologous bone marrow-derived mesenchymal stem cells delivered by transendocardial injection in patients with ischemic cardiomyopathy: the PO-SEIDON randomized trial," The Journal of the American Medical Association, vol. 308, no. 22, pp. 2369–2379, 2012.

4. R. Bolli, A. R. Chugh, D. D'Amario et al., "Cardiac stem cells in patients with ischaemic cardiomyopathy (SCIPIO): initial results of a randomised phase 1 trial," The Lancet, vol. 378, no. 9806, pp. 1847–1857, 2011

5. A. R. Chugh, G. M. Beache, J. H. Loughran et al., "Administra-tion of cardiac stem cells in patients with ischemic cardiomyopathy: the SCIPIO trial: surgical aspects and interim analysis of myocardial function and viability by magnetic resonance," Circulation, vol. 126, no. 11, supplement 1, pp. S54–S64, 2012

6. Lins Kusterer LEF (2011) Oral Diseases and Liver Pre and Post-Transplantation Disorders. J Transplant Technol Res S1: 001.

7.   Vitin AA, Martay K, Vater Y, Dembo G, Maziarz M (2010) Effects of
      Vasoactive Agents on Blood Loss and Transfusion Requirements During
      Pre-Reperfusion Stages of the Orthotopic Liver Transplantation. J Anesthe
      Clinic Res 1: 104

8.   Berzoff J, Swantkowski J, Cohen LM. 2008. Developing a renal supportive
      care team from the voices of patients, families, and palliative care staff. Palliat
      Support Care 6(2):133-139.

9.   Imberti B, Morigi M, Tomasoni S, Rota C, Corna D, Longaretti L, Rottoli
      D, Valsecchi F, Benigni A, Wang J, Abbate M, Zoja C, Remuzzi G. 2007.
      Insulin-like growth factor-1 sustains stem cell mediated renal repair. J Am
      Soc Nephrol 18(11):2921-2928

10.   Niewoehner D. Structure-function relationships: the pathophysiology of
      airflow obstruction. In: Stockley R, Rnnard S. Rabe K, Celli B, eds. Chronic
      Obstructive Pulmonary Disease. Hoboken, NJ: Blackwell, 2007: 3-19.

11.   Fernando J Martinez, James F Donohue, Stephen I Rennard. The future of
      chronic obstructive pulmonary disease treatment-difficulties of and barriers
      to drug development. Lancet 2011; 378: 1027-37

9

OTHER USES OF STEM CELL THERAPY

Stem cell therapy research and its incorporation into mainstream medicine has really changed the whole treatment spectrum for a variety of diseases, particularly degenerative ones.

On the other hand, stem cells have also made their way into the fields of aesthetics cosmetology, dermatology and plastic surgery. Its implications are unlimited and seems to be an exciting feat. Although we won't be diving deep into this aspect, this chapter will be walking you through the basics of some other uses of stem cell therapy.

The only reason we will not be exploring these areas or uses of stem cell therapy is because they delve more into the aesthetical side of medicine. Our focus is more on ushering stem cells into mainstream medicine so it can be opted as a first line of treatment for degenerative conditions and/or diseases.

They aren't called 'master cells' for nothing. Statistics

compiled by the National Institute of Health suggest that an approximate 1 billion dollars are spent on stem cell research per year, and with good reason. Millions of stem cells are harvested from different sites of the body and isolated in the lab. Here they are manipulated, pricked and pronged to yield the required specialized cells.

Stem cells show immense promise in treating a wide range of diseases, injuries, and other health conditions. They are currently used for facial fat transfer, gluteal and breast augmentation, skin rejuvenation, healing of burns and wounds, reversal of baldness and cellulite treatment. [1]

However, since stem cells differentiate into highly specialized cells (depending upon the tissue they are harvested from), the same treatment is not likely to work for conditions affecting other organs unless the stem cells are manipulated in the lab first. Induced pluripotent stem cells are being studied by scientists to produce specific cells by meticulously integrating them with complex instructions. If the instructions go haywire after transplantation it may cause an overgrowth of cells and lead to tumor formation. [2]

Here are some other non-conventional implementations of stem cell therapies:

Breast Augmentation

Bust size has always been a social taboo in most societies. It has also been much talked about because of the potential adverse effects of implants. Initially, silicone implants were used, which proved to be unhealthy and led to multiple corrective surgeries afterwards. The more recent approach has been saline and cohesive silicone implants. Now, the talk of today is stem cell transplantation. It is also referred to as natural implantation as stem cells are taken from the host's adipose tissue and transplanted into the breast tissue of the same person.

Adipose tissue of any part of the body can be accessed, but the most common and preferred site is belly fat. This results in an added advantage of fat removal from stomach region. This method has proven to be much safer and free from complications that tend to occur with unnatural implants. It also defines the breasts aesthetically i.e. they look and feel more natural. With silicone implants, capsular contraction can occur which causes the breast tissue around the implant to harden. This is not the case with stem cell breast augmentation. The only real limitation however is the cost. Since it is not commercially available as mainstream therapy, it is quite expensive. [3]

Cosmetology

Plastic surgery has become a flooding field in terms of facial 'beautification', especially when it comes to facelifts, nose jobs and pouty lips. Patients mainly aim to look younger. While this may be achieved to a certain extent, it definitely doesn't look natural.

The effects of ageing are most prominent on the face, particularly around the eyes, nose and lips. Certain creases and lines become more prominent and later on take the form of wrinkles. With the advent of stem cell therapy, much research is carried out about the ageing process on the face itself. Now, facelifts are being done using stem cells which leaves the face looking more natural and youthful. This procedure has reduced the need for Botox injections and soft-tissue fillers.

Stem cells are also being used for stem cell rejuvenation. This is a technique in which stem cells are harvested from the fat of the belly or medial thigh region and implanted into the facial tissue under the influence of certain growth factors. They induce the skin and under-lying fatty tissue to generate their own cells as well. [4]

Hair Growth

Hair loss has never really been considered as a medical condition. Hence it is mostly treated by conventional methods. Hair tonics, solutions and home-made remedies don't always do the trick.

Several forms of hair loss affect men and women. The two most common types of hair loss are:

- Age-related alopecia: This type of hair loss comes naturally with age and is inevitable.

- Alopecia Areata. This is an auto immune condition in which immune cells attack hair follicles and large locks of hair falls off.

- Androgenetic Alopecia. This too affects both men and women and begins at an early age. This condition has a genetic predisposition.

At present there are only two drugs used for hair loss that are approved by the FDA. The more commonly prescribed one is

'Minidoxil'. This causes a great deal of hormonal imbalance in females hence its use is cautioned and should not be considered without a doctor's advice and supervision.

Besides drugs, hair transplants are also used as a treatment modality for hair loss. Despite its success, it still remains expensive and the regeneration of new hair follicles is challenging. [5]

The advent of stem cell therapy however, has changed the way hair loss is being treated. There are various methods but the principle is the same. Mesenchymal stem cells within the hair follicles are being used to stimulate growth of new hair.

A study performed in China used stem cells that resided within dermal papilla cells. An optimized microenvironment was created in which the cells were exposed to fibroblast growth factor-2, an important culture nutrient that enhances hair induction and proliferation.

Scientists have also found a way to induce growth of hair stem cells by manipulating macrophages into reactivating hair follicles. This trait of macrophages was discovered by accident during a study in which mice were given anti-inflammatory drugs and hair growth was a side effect of it. They found that the macrophages stimulated stem cells in hair follicles and induced hair growth in non-inflamed skin. [6]

Skin Rejuvenation

Your skin is perhaps the most important organ. It is underrated and under stated in terms of care, function and significance. But when it comes to looking fresh and maintaining a natural buoyancy of the skin, the market is full of products that promise to rejuvenate and regenerate new skin cells helping your skin look flawless.

The advent of stem cells has taken the world by storm. They are being used in all sorts of therapies, particularly regenerative ones. Several studies have been carried out in which the regenerative potential and safety of stem cells has been scrutinized. Although most stem cell therapies are still highly experimental, they still offer promise to patients in need.

Stem cells are popular because of their biology. Their hallmark characteristic is that they can develop into any cell lineage. It has also been found that stem cells change their properties throughout life to meet the demands of change that occur during growth and regeneration. [7]

It is a well-known fact that skin cells shed and regenerate almost on a daily basis. The dead cells come to the surface of the skin while new skin cells develop underneath.

Skin care brands are seeking out stem cells and hoping that they prove to be as useful in the cosmetic industry as they are in Medicine. Most skin care products either contain plant based stem cells or human stem cells derived from unfertilized eggs. Thus it is always better to check the specifics of the brand before using it.

The mechanism of action of stem cells works on two basic components:

- Growth factors which facilitate cell growth and cell division

- Proteins which regulate cell division

Plant-derived stem cells don't work in the same way as human stem cells. Human stem cells stimulate the growth of new epidermal cells. This not only thickens the skin but rejuvenates it as well. There is no scientific evidence indicating that plant-based stem cells function in the same way. Having said this, plant-based products which come from rich anti-oxidant fruits or plants exhibit free radical fighting properties. [8]

An important tip before buying stem cell containing skin care products is to check the ingredient list on the back to confirm the quantity of the active ingredient. If stem cell is placed on the top of the list that most probably means that it is present as a chief ingredient.

Anti Aging

Statistics reveal that millions are spent on the production of anti-aging products every year. Anti-aging products or therapies delay the degeneration process of the skin and its stroma.

The natural ageing process stretches the skin. Its elasticity is reduced and collagen distribution is altered. Sun exposure is also a significant factor that speeds up the physiological process of ageing. One or a combination of the above mentioned processes result in the formation of wrinkles and premature skin folds.

Apparently the phenomenon of ageing is a plethora of molecular and chemical reactions. Therefore, anti-ageing therapies will only be effective if they impact one of those mechanisms.

One of the processes that is targeted by anti-ageing products/therapies is collagen remodeling or collagen synthesis. Laser treatment, for instance, stimulates the formation of collagen type

I and type III. Collagen formation is also affected by growth factors and cytokines. These factors act on dermal fibroblasts thereby inciting collagen synthesis. This is where stem cells come in. Stem cells that are capable of producing these growth factors and cytokines hold promise for anti-ageing therapies. [7]

Even though there is still plenty of room for improvement, it still seems to be a promising area for research. A research was conducted on mice which showed that Adult Stem Cells were able to reverse the effects of UV induced wrinkles by secreting factors that activated dermal fibroblasts. Scientists are working on providing an optimal environment for transplanted stem cells to function in.

For instance, when an enriching microenvironment is provided, autologous MSCs along with hyaluronic acid have been shown to fill in deep skin folds in the face, resulting in an increased skin tone and fewer lines of expression.

It seems like stem cells comprise of an almost infinite potential unleashing a new discovery at every turn.

REFERENCES

1.   Stem Cells in Aesthetic Medicine. (2011, December 07). Retrieved from The American Academy of Anti-ageing medicine: http://www.a4m.com/las-vegas-2011-stem-cells-in-aesthetic-medicine.html

2.   Nine Things. (2015). Retrieved from A closer look at stem cells: http://www.closerlookatstemcells.org/stem-cells-and-medicine/nine-things-to-know-about-stem-cell-treatments

3.   Murnaghan, I. (2016, December 03). Breast Implants from Stem Cells. Retrieved from Explore Stem Cells: http://www.explorestemcells.co.uk/breast-implants-from-stem-cells.html

4.   The Stem Cell Facelift. (2009). Retrieved from Stem Cell Facelift: http://www.stemcellfacelift.us/The-Stem-Cell-Facelift.html

5.   Howson, S. (2015, December 22). Re-seeding hairlines with stem cells. Retrieved from Chemistry World: https://www.chemistryworld.com/news/re-seeding-hairlines-with-stem-cells/9281.article

6.   Dovey, D. (2014, December 23). Cure For Baldness? Spanish Scientists Use Stem Cells To Restore Hair Growth. Retrieved from MedicalDaily: http://www.medicaldaily.com/cure-baldness-spanish-scientists-use-stem-cells-restore-hair-growth-315446

7.   McArdle, A. (2014). The Role of Stem Cells in Aesthetic Surgery. Plastic Reconstructive Surgery, 193-200.

8.   5 thing you need to know about stem cells in skin care. (2013, June 19). Retrieved from fabfitfun: https://fabfitfun.com/magazine/stem-cells-in-skin-care/

10

PHARMACEUTICAL DISPUTE

This chapter was difficult to write because pharmaceutical research is rare in Mexico. There are clinical trials done in this country, but are not preferred over the headquarters of big pharma in America. The following information is based on the U.S. pharmaceutical industry and our perception from continuously attending several medical conferences in the country.

In the past couple of years, big names in the pharmaceutical industry have had to bear the brunt against several allegations and claims that it has in fact become more of a 'business' in the context of corporate interest and gain.

With an increase in the burden of health issues worldwide, the production of drugs has increased exponentially and so have the prices. According to a reputable news report, drug prices in the United States has been skyrocketing due to certain government regulations. The big pharmaceuticals aren't being opposed by their competitors either resulting in a huge increment in the amount spent on prescription drugs in the U.S. Currently, each person spends around $900 on prescription drugs alone as compared to an average of $400 per person across 19 other industrialized nations across the world. In fact, it comes as no surprise when prescription drugs add up to 17% overall healthcare expenses. [1]

This rise in drug expenses doesn't only affect those without insurance. Since insurance companies aren't 'allowed' to oppose the highly priced drugs or negotiate, they have started to incorporate the costlier drugs into higher levels of medical coverage. This eventually results in a larger co-pay for each prescription.

So, what favors this over pricing of medicines by drug manufacturers? An instructor at Harvard Medical School and the Harvard T.H. Chan School of Public Health in Boston calls is "market exclusivity". Drugs that are selective and more targeted are the ones that can get away with being pricier than the rest. Unfortunately, this monopolization of drugs prevents people from sticking to the medicines. The more expensive the drugs are, the harder it is for patients to comply with them.

The following are just some examples of how the price of potentially lifesaving drugs has gone up in the recent past:

- The Epipen has gone up from $57 to more than $500 over a period of just nine years. According to Forbes, this has put allergy patients at a higher risk as their access has to epipens has been limited.

- A fairly common and cheap drug, even in the developing countries of the world in the anti-malaria pill. Its price has increased by 5000% in just one year.

The once $13 pill now costs over $700.

- The hepatitis pill made some news a couple of years back as a means of ground-breaking treatment, especially since the disease prevalence was increasing worldwide. It is a whopping $1000 per pill. It costs less than half in some of the developing countries where Hepatitis C is an epidemic.

WHAT DOES THE FDA HAVE TO DO WITH IT?

Once the FDA approves a drug for commercial use, it sets a period of 'market exclusivity' that can be anywhere from 5 to 12 years. During this time, another low-priced generic version of the medicine cannot be sold.

How do the pharmaceutical companies maintain the price of a drug for so long?

As the period of exclusivity for a drug comes to an end, the drug manufacturing company will make a minor change in the on-going selling drug and then promote the newer version as being more beneficial than the previous one. Patients who are now being prescribed the 'new and improved' version will not go for the generic one.

THE FDA AND STEM CELL THERAPY

Stem cell therapy holds so much promise in the future and can revolutionize a wide spectrum of diseases and conditions, if it was accepted as a mainstream therapy by the FDA. The FDA's Center for Biologics Evaluation and Research (CBER) regulates the transfer of human cells, tissues, and cellular and tissue-based products (HCT/P) into a human recipient. Stem cells are considered HCT/Ps and are regulated by the FDA to prevent transmission of communicable disease.

The debate is that mesenchymal stem cells (MSCs) could be autologous and therefore, will only affect the person they are taken from. Autologous MSCs are presented as biological drugs, but the FDA views them as human and cell based 'products'. The FDA maintains that any process that includes culturing, expansion, and added growth factors or antibiotics requires regulation because the process constitutes significant manipulation.

So doctors using autologous stem cells are forced to follow the manufacturing standards as for any regular pharmaceutical product. The whole process can become quite complicated. To avoid limitations and hassle, such doctors claim that autologous stem cells without manipulation are not a concern for the FDA.

The efficacy and safety of stem cell based therapy has always been an area of great concern for the FDA. They say that stem cells when manipulated outside of their natural environment can at any stage be of potential danger to the recipient. According to the FDA, stem cell therapy may cause tumor formation, immune reactions and growth of unwanted tissue. [2]

Things get more complicated when a company manipulates/ prepares the stem cell units in order to make them appropriate for use in allogenic procedures. Once the stem cells are infused to another patient other than the donor, the risks mentioned above are more likely to occur.

On one hand, the future of Stem cells by manipulation, cell

production, induction of pluripotent cells, and embryonic stem cells is bright for the general population, but the FDA still deems it risky. On the other hand many people are trying to explain that there are other stem cell procedures where no manipulation is needed and the risks are minimum using autologous stem cells. It is worth mentioning again that fresh autologous stem cells most of the times have the benefit of high viability, minimal manipulation, high level of activity, without the risk of immune rejection, dormant medical conditions, etc.

As long as autologous and allogenic stem cells are reviewed under the same umbrella holding both to the same standard, there is no way to move forward. The goal for stem cell treatment has to be the same whether it's for a specific case or for a mass population. Authorities will have a very hard time approving stem cells in general; it will take years to approve specifics one by one (specific stem cells for specific medical conditions).

We can see that stem cell therapy is becoming a real possibility of treatment and is a different path when compared to traditional medication and treatment.

These are just some of the challenges that need to be overcome by researchers and experts of this field. There are ongoing debates and cases with the FDA for this matter.

REFERENCES

1. THOMPSON, D. (2016). What's behind the sharp rise in prescription drug prices? CBS News.

2. Reisman, M. (2014). Stem Cell Therapy: a Look at Current Research, Regulations, and Remaining Hurdles. Pharmacy and Therapeutics, 846-847, 854-857.

11

WHEN TO CONSIDER STEM CELL THERAPY

Over the recent years, stem cell therapy has shown great promise in the treatment of a wide spectrum of conditions and diseases. The discovery of stem cells has been ground breaking and has revolutionized the way diseases are assessed, particularly degenerative ones.

For instance, they have been used for tissue grafts in the skin and the surface of the eyes, as well as for retinal regeneration and to increase the efficiency of internal organs. Blood forming stem cells have also saved thousands of children with leukemia. Stem cells have further been explored and their potential has been eye opening. The characteristic trait of stem cells is that of differentiation potential. They are able to develop into almost any cell type.

There are various different types of stem cells as well (depending upon their source). Stem cells are found in:

- Bone marrow

- Adipose tissue

- Dental pulp

- Placenta

- Umbilical cord

- Amniotic fluid

There are many other sources, but the ones mentioned above are more common.

The various applications of stem cells are still being investigated in clinical trials as they do have their limitations. Evidence collected from the clinical trials determines whether a proposed treatment is safe or not. In some conditions, stem cell treatment is safe, effective and better than existing treatments with minimal side effects.

It is very important to read up on stem cell therapy and discuss your concerns with your physician to find out what is right for you. Evidence based medicine usually makes the decision easier. However, if you have a condition, which has unproven or experimental treatment you may feel like there is nothing to lose if other treatment options have failed. In this case, it is always better to consult an expert for advice to avoid unwanted complications or long term health effects. Consider the risks and benefits, but be careful of input from family and friends. Sometimes their talks are based upon rumors or distorted stories, without proper or real knowledge. It is always important to take the proper advice from a legitimate source.

Most people with degenerative conditions are good candidates for stem cell therapy. Degenerative conditions refer to those diseases in which there is constant wear and tear of affected tissue. Mainstream medicine is mostly aimed at supportive and palliative treatment for short term and temporary relief of symptoms.

Stem cell therapy, however, aims at regenerative healing. The stem cell's ability to divide and form a specific cell type allows targeted therapy. The damaged cells are replaced by new and healthy cells. Be cautious of the cells that are manipulated for differentiation in a lab before transplant, as they supposedly tend to yield favorable results. However, if they're not 'directed' properly, it may result in overgrowth of cells and tumors when injected into the patient.

It is very important to understand the pathophysiology of your disease before opting for treatment, particularly stem cell therapy. A better comprehension of the cause and effects of your condition will help you make the best choice. The stem cell therapy is tailored according to your condition so it can provide the desired results.

There is a long list of conditions that can potentially be treated with stem cell therapy. However, following are some of the more common ones:

Pluripotent stem cells are being used widely in clinical trials and research. They have shown success:

- Neurological conditions like Parkinson's disease, Alzheimer's, Motor Neuron Disease and Huntington's Disease

- Macular degeneration

- Spinal Cord injury

- Myocardial Infarction

- Diabetes mellitus

- Degenerative liver disease

- Multiple sclerosis

- Arthritis

- Lung disorders

- Memory loss

- Allergies and sinusitis

- Stroke

PREPARATION BEFORE STEM CELL TRANSPLANT

A little mental preparation never hurts anyone. It always helps to know beforehand what you'll be expecting. This will not only reduce the stress, but being foresighted and positive when going in has shown to lead to a speedy recovery on the way out. Preparation of the body is important; therefore, recommendations are suggested for a better engraftment and development of the cells.

ASSESSMENT AND DIAGNOSTICS

When doctors consider that stem cell therapy is the way to go for a patient, they carry out a detailed assessment before the procedure. While each procedure is different in terms of modifying it to the condition in question, there are some fundamental basics that are covered. A series of pre-transplant diagnostic tests are done to make sure that the patient is physically and mentally prepared.

Some or all of the following tests may be prescribed:

- Complete medical history and physical examination

- Routine blood tests

- Tests for certain viruses (hepatitis, herpes and HIV)

- Bone marrow biopsy

- Human leukocyte antigen (HLA) A protein found on the surface of all cells, including white blood cells (leukocytes) and platelets, that plays a role in the immune system's response to foreign substances

- CT/MRI

- Electrocardiogram (ECG) and echocardiogram (Echo) to check the heart functions

- Chest x-ray and pulmonary function test (PFT) to measure how well the lungs are working, how much air the lungs can hold, how quickly air moves in and out of the lungs, and how much oxygen is taken in and how much carbon dioxide is given off to check lung function

In case of an allogenic transplant, donor matching plays a very important role. The closest match is that of an identical twin since both have the same HLA. However, if that's not the case then the immediate family members like siblings and parents are tested first. These cases are the precise ones when stored umbilical cord blood becomes handy.

HLA typing is done by a blood test. At least 6-10 antigens have to match. There is a 25% chance of a sibling having a match to the recipient. The more siblings there are, the higher is the chance of finding a match. If a sibling match is not found, then the extended family is reached like aunts, uncles, and cousins.

HARVESTING STEM CELLS

As previously discussed, 'harvesting' refers to the collection or extraction of stem cells. Days in advance of the harvesting, the patient could be put through a technique of a series of injections of medication to stimulate production of stem cells in his/her system. This is the time when healthy cells are in abundance.

NUTRITION

Is recommended that a patient gets their stem cell therapy with a healthy body, therefore consultation with a dietician is necessary so that he/she can carry out a nutritional assessment to make sure the recipient has an adequate intake of healthy food. It is important for the patient to be eating well at least 2 weeks before the procedure and 2 weeks after the procedure. An overall improved state of health will only increase the endurance of the patient. It is often said that while the stem cells may be a booster, the nutrition is a sustainer.

It's like a balancing act as any disease and its treatment can affect nutrition as well. Since feeling sick often leads to loss of appetite or desire to eat, it is important to prepare the body before treatment begins.

Nutrition therapy is advised for some patients, which guide them to consume the right kinds of food and liquids to keep a healthy weight, boost the immune system, and keep the body systems healthy. Adequate amount of calories and protein are important, especially in patients suffering from diabetes.

Certain medicines can also be used to correct the nutritional deficiencies. For instance:

- Appetite stimulants

- Medicines to help digestion

- Anti-emetics

- Medicines to help with nausea

- Laxatives to help with constipation

The structure of stem cells is made up of protein. The units of a protein are amino acids. Research suggests that polyphenols and amino acids are prominent in aiding stem cell transplants. [1]

Like all other cells of the human body, stem cells also age and lose their ability to repair and regenerate. Good nutrition can delay this ageing and rather increase the production and proliferation of healthy stem cells. The healthier the stem cells you have, the slower you will age. Evidence shows that the infusion of stem cells in anti-ageing treatments are increasing by the day.

The fact of the matter is that the diet recommendation throughout stem cell therapy is actually pretty much the same as the one to get healthier under normal circumstances. Now, because the effects of poor eating aren't seen immediately, one often fails to realize its downfalls.

Stem cells need adequate nutrition to thrive. The basics are to cut down on sugar, excess refined carbs, reduce calories, cut out smoking and practice exercise. Most of the degenerative conditions, such as orthopedic ailments and diabetes, which are to be treated by stem cell therapy could have been prevented in the first place naturally by restricting diet and eating healthy.

There are well laid out and thought out diet plans for different conditions in the nutrition chapter of this book. Here are some general tips to follow:

- Fresh fruits and vegetables are advised, but caution should be taken that they must be fresh and well washed. Not bruised or with broken skin.

- Raw or rare cooked meat, fish, poultry, and eggs should be avoided. Meat should be well cooked and eggs should be cooked completely.

- Leftovers older than 3 days should not be consumed.

- Avoid sharing food or drinks with sick persons, even if they are slightly symptomatic, including family members.

- Dairy products must be pasteurized.

- Proper hand washing is essential as well as keeping handles, knobs, and cutting boards clean and sanitized.

- Avoid condiments and preserved food when eating out.

- Avoid bad smelling foods.

- Refrain from eating raw vegetables when eating out.

- Avoid eating from street vendors.

There is additional nutritional information in Chapter 15 where you can find lifestyle tips and recipies for healthy living.

HYDRATION

By far this would have to be the most important health aspect. The human body is made up of 75% water. Staying hydrated is extremely important for normal function from the cellular level to the organic level. Good hydration replenishes and revitalizes the blood, purges toxins out of your system, and improves kidney function, hence, excretes several unwanted elements via urine.

When obtaining bone marrow stem cells, having a good hydrated system comes with advantages. Bone marrow has a lower viscosity, therefore, flows easier inside the bone and conduits. Easier flow causes less discomfort to the patient during aspiration. Higher volume of bone marrow is achieved in less time. It is a win-win situation for the patient and for the medical team.

A good hydrated environment at the cellular level ensures cellular homeostasis and electrolyte balance. It provides a functional environment for the healthy stem cells to thrive and proliferate without resistance. This means easier regeneration of the bone marrow volume aspirated during a procedure.

EXERCISE

Proper exercise before your treatment is recommended. It will limit the inflammation in your body, improve sleep, lower your blood pressure, and help you lose weight. Twenty-four hours post-treatment, when you feel like you're regaining your energy, light to moderate intensity of exercise would be very beneficial. Exercise has an immense benefit to your mental health and boosts your confidence like no other. It also improves blood flow in areas of the body, which otherwise have scarce blood flow. Areas with the dampened blood flow have a higher chance of inflammation. Inflammation actually restricts the stem cells to exert their maximum potential.

SLEEP

Catching up on sleep is also essential to maintain a healthy mind and body. At least 8 hours of sleep is recommended and the 'golden hours' are said to be from 10 pm to 6 am. If you aren't sleeping to a minimum of 8 hours, it could result in an increase in blood pressure, weight, insulin resistance, and body inflammation.

It is normal to feel tired after treatment. A lot of stress flows through your body and the increase in activity of your metabolism causes fatigue. Plan a good rest after any medical intervention.

NATURAL ANTI-INFLAMMATORIES AND SUPPLEMENTS

Some experts suggest that over the counter anti-inflammatories or supplements should not be taken right before and after a treatment procedure because the patient is more vulnerable to side effects during this period. Having said this, there are certain natural ingredients out there, which are preferred such as curcumin (derivative of turmeric), fish oils, omega 3 fatty acids, and glucosamine. Peppermint oil, eucalyptus, lavender, etc. can be taken to reduce stress and inflammation.

The following is a list of foods to avoid, as they can enhance inflammation:

- High amount of Carbohydrates

- Energy drinks

- Artificial sweeteners (aspartame, sucralose)

- Oils: corn, soybean, safflower, vegetable

- Dairy products should be limited

- Spicy food

PRACTICAL PLAN

Plan ahead, this is a very stressful time for the patient and family members. The anxiety of the procedure is not the only thing that crosses one's mind. Job absence leads to work accumulation, traveling is always a hassle, and if you're a parent, then one of your concerns will be the care your kids until getting back home. It's always better to involve close family and friends as they want to feel useful as well.

Plan out important and eventful days ahead to ensure that the pre-existing commitments are fulfilled. Take some time off work. Give your boss and colleagues a heads up before your procedure started, so they can fill in a replacement for you.

Get your finances in order, so the last thing you have to worry about is the last minute money problems.

WHAT SHOULD YOU BRING TO THE MEDICAL FACILITY?

Usually stem cell therapy takes only a few hours over a series of days. Most likely overnight stay is at home or at a hotel. So pack accordingly.

There are only a few things to bring to the medical facility:

- Medical records, recent and any past records, related to your current condition.

- Some sort of identification, when traveling abroad don't forget your citizenship documents.

- Medications for the length of the trip, and some extras in case you need to stay longer.

- Inform your nurse if you have an allergy to any foods or medications.

- Insurance card

- Payment form

- Relaxed dress code: It is really helpful to feel comfortable during a medical treatment; loose clothes and comfy shoes are a must.

- Some facilities are very busy and medical teams can get back up with emergency surgeries, so a good book or electronic device is a nice companion.

REFERENCES

1. *ALS Fact Sheet.* (n.d.). Retrieved from National Institute of Neurological Disorders and Stroke: https://www.ninds.nih.gov/Disorders/Patient-Caregiver-Education/Fact-Sheets/Amyotrophic-Lateral-Sclerosis-ALS-Fact-Sheet

2. Augello, A. (2007). Cell therapy using allogeneic bone marrow mesenchymal stem cells prevents tissue damage in collagen-induced arthritis. *Arthritis and Rheumatology* , 1175–1186.

3.   Ballabio, F. L. (2009). Stem cell therapy in stroke. *Cellular and Molecular Life Sciences* , 757–772.

4.   Behjati, M. (2013). Suggested indications of clinical practice guideline for stem cell-therapy in cardiovascular diseases: A stepwise appropriate use criteria for regeneration therapy. *ARYA Atherosclerosis* , 306-310.

5.   *Bone Marrow Aspiration and Biopsy.* (2015). Retrieved from Cancer.Net: http://www.cancer.net/navigating-cancer-care/diagnosing-cancer/tests-and-procedures/bone-marrow-aspiration-and-biopsy

6.   Boseley, S. (2015). *First UK patient receives stem cell treatment to cure loss of vision.* London: The Guardian.

7.   Centeno, C. (2016, July 18). *8 Ways to increase stem cell health.* Retrieved from Regennex: http://www.regenexx.com/8-ways-improve-your-stem-cells-prior-treatment/

8.   *Chronic liver disease: how could regenerative medicine help?* (2016). Retrieved from Swiss Medica: http://www.startstemcells.com/liver-cirrhosis-treatment.html

9.   Cras, A. (2015). Update on mesenchymal stem cell-based therapy in lupus and scleroderma. *Arthritis Research and Therapy* , 301.

10.   *Diabetes: how could stem cells help?* (2015, November 09). Retrieved from Euro Stem Cell: http://www.eurostemcell.org/factsheet/diabetes-how-could-stem-cells-help

11.   Elvis, A. M. (2011). Ozone therapy: A clinical review. *Journal of Natural Science, Biology and Medicine* , 66–70.

12.   *Exercise triggers stem cells in muscle.* (2012, February 6). Retrieved from Science Daily: https://www.sciencedaily.com/releases/2012/02/120206143944.htm

13.   *Fat Stem Cell Therapy.* (2015). Retrieved from Infinite Horizons Medical Center: http://www.fatstemcelltherapy.com/procedure/

14.   *Handout on Health: Rheumatoid Arthritis.* (2016, February). Retrieved from National Institute of Arthritis and Musculoskeletal and Skin Diseases: https://www.niams.nih.gov/health_info/rheumatic_disease/#ra_5

15.   Helwick, C. (2013, May 22). *Stem Cell Transplantation Halts Crohn's Disease.* Retrieved from Medscape: http://www.medscape.com/viewarticle/804570

16.   Ichim, T. E. (2007). Stem Cell Therapy for Autism. *Journal of Translational Medicine* , 5:30.

17.   Imran Ullah, *. R. (2015). Human mesenchymal stem cells - current trends
       and future prospective. *Bioscience Reports* , 35 (2).

18.   Jr., W. C. (2017). *Symptoms of psriatic arthritis* . Retrieved from Medicine Net:
       http://www.medicinenet.com/psoriatic_arthritis/page3.htm

19.   Kehr, W. (2016, October 3). *Ozone Cancer Treatments.* Retrieved from Cancer
       Tutor: https://www.cancertutor.com/ozone/

20.   Kim, J.-H. (2002). Dopamine neurons derived from embryonic stem cells
       function in an animal model of Parkinson's disease. *nature, International weekly
       journal of Science* , 50-56.

21.   Kramerov, A. A. (2015). Stem cell therapies in the treatment of diabetic reti-
       nopathy and keratopathy. *Experimental Biology and Medicine* , 559–568.

22.   lajimi, A. A. (2013). Feasibility of Cell Therapy in Multiple Sclerosis: A Sys-
       tematic Review of 83 Studies. *International Journal of Hematology-Oncology and
       Stem Cell Research* , 15-33.

23.   Latham, E. (2016, July 22). *Hyperbaric oxygen therapy.* Retrieved from Med-
       scape: http://emedicine.medscape.com/article/1464149-overview

24.   Lunn, J. S. (2011). Stem Cell Technology for Neurodegenerative Diseases.
       Ann Neurology , 353–361.

25.   Martin R, M. H. (January 24, 2017). Assessment of Patients With Multiple
       Sclerosis (MS). *National Institute of Neurological Disorders and Stroke (NINDS)* .

26.   Mazzini, L. (2008). Stem cell treatment in Amyotrophic Lateral Sclerosis.
       Journal of the Neurological Sciences , 78–83.

27.   McKhann GM, K. D. (2011). The diagnosis of dementia due to Alzheimer's
       disease: Recommendations from the National Institute on Aging-Alzheimer's
       Association workgroups on diagnostic guidelines for Alzheimer's disease.
       Alzheimer's and Dementia , 263-269.

28.   *Motor Neuron Disease Information.* (n.d.). Retrieved from National Institute of
       Neurological Diseases and Stroke: https://www.ninds.nih.gov/Disorders/
       All-Disorders/Motor-Neuron-Diseases-Information-Page

29.   Munoz J, S. N. (2014). umbilical cord blood transplantation: past, present,
       and future. *Stem Cells Transl Med* , 1435-1443.

30.   OM, A.-S. (2011). Stem cell therapy for Alzheimer's disease. *CNS Neurological
       DIsroders Drug Targets* , 459-85.

31. Patricia A. Zuk, *. M. (2002). Human Adipose Tissue Is a Source of Multipotent Stem Cells. *Molecular Biology of the Cell* , 4279–4295.

32. Prof Vincenzo Silani, M. (2004). Stem-cell therapy for amyotrophic lateral sclerosis. *The Lancet* , 200–202.

33. Richard K. Burt, M., Roumen Balabanov, M., Xiaoqiang Han, M., & al, e. (2015). Association of Nonmyeloablative Hematopoietic Stem Cell Transplantation With Neurological Disability in Patients With Relapsing-Remitting Multiple Sclerosis. *Journal of the American Medical Association (JAMA)*. , 275-284.

34. Riordan, N. (2016). *Stem Cell Therapy* . Retrieved from stem cell Institute: https://www.cellmedicine.com/stem-cell-therapy-for-multiple-sclerosis-3/

35. Shroff, G. (2016). Human Embryonic Stem Cell Therapy in Crohn's Disease: A Case Report. *The American Journal of Case Reports* , 124–128.

36. *Signs and Symptoms of ASD.* (n.d.). Retrieved from Centres for Disease Control and Prevention: https://www.cdc.gov/ncbddd/autism/signs.html

37. *Stem cell harvest procedure.* (2016). Retrieved from Non Hodgkin Lymphoma Cyberfamily: http://www.nhlcyberfamily.org/treatments/collection.htm#-methods

38. *Stem Cell Therapy* . (2016). Retrieved from Stem Cell Institute: https://www.cellmedicine.com/stem-cell-therapy-for-osteoarthritis/

39. *Stem Cell Therapy and spinal cord injury.* (2016). Retrieved from Stem cell institute: https://www.cellmedicine.com/stem-cell-therapy-for-spinal-cord-injury/

40. *Stem Cell/Bone Marrow Collection.* (n.d.). Retrieved from Blood and Marrow transplant information network: http://www.bmtinfonet.org/before/stem-cellmarrowharvest

41. Sung, S. M. (2015). *Remission of Psoriasis 13 Years After Autologous Stem Cell Transplant.* Parsippany, NJ, USA: Frontline Medical Communications Inc.

42. Terskikh AV, E. M. (2001). From hematopoiesis to neuropoiesis: evidence of overlapping genetic programs. *Proc Natl Acad Sci U S A* , 7934-9.

43. *Tests and Procedures. Hyperbaric Oxygen Therapy.* (1998-2016). Retrieved from Mayo Clinic: http://www.mayoclinic.org/tests-procedures/hyperbaric-oxygen-therapy/basics/why-its-done/prc-20019167

44. *The Bone Marrow Harvest Procedure.* (1995-2016). Retrieved from Cleveland Clinic: http://my.clevelandclinic.org/health/treatments_and_procedures/hic_Bone_Marrow_and_Transplantation/hic-bone-marrow-harvest-procedure

45. *The Importance of Nutrition before Bone Marrow or Stem Cell Transplant.* (2012). Retrieved from Bone Marrow Transplant at Angeles Health International: http://www.bonemarrowmx.com/the-importance-of-nutrition-before-bone-marrow-transplant-or-stem-cell-transplant/

46. *Traumatic Brain Injury.* (2016, October 11). Retrieved from Medline Plus: https://medlineplus.gov/traumaticbraininjury.html#cat95

47. *Turning Stem Cells into Insulin-Producing Cells.* (2016). Retrieved from Diabetes Research Institute Foundation: https://www.diabetesresearch.org/stem-cells

48. Wang, S. (2010). Non-Invasive Stem Cell Therapy in a Rat Model for Retinal Degeneration and Vascular Pathology. *PLOS one* .

49. Weiss, D. J. (2014). Current Status of Stem Cells and Regenerative Medicine in Lung Biology and Diseases. *Stem Cells* , 16–25.

50. Weiss, J. N. (2015). Stem Cell Ophthalmology Treatment Study (SCOTS) for retinal and optic nerve diseases: a preliminary report. *Neural regeneration research* , 982–988.

51. Weiss, M. L. (2005). Human Umbilical Cord Matrix Stem Cells: Preliminary Characterization and Effect of Transplantation in a Rodent Model of Parkinson's Disease. *Stem Cells* .

52. *What are the Causes of TBI?* (2001). Retrieved from Traumatic Brain Injury. com: http://www.traumaticbraininjury.com/understanding-tbi/what-are-the-causes-of-tbi/

53. *What is Psoriatic arthritis.* (2017). Retrieved from Arhritis Research UK: http://www.arthritisresearchuk.org/arthritis-information/conditions/psoriatic-arthritis/causes.aspx

54. Woods, A. C. (2006). Amelioration of severe psoriasis with psoriatic arthritis for 20 years after allogeneic haematopoietic stem cell transplantation. *Annals of the Rheumatic Diseases* , 65(5): 697.

55. Xu, J. (2012). Allogeneic mesenchymal stem cell treatment alleviates experimental and clinical Sjögren syndrome. *Blood* , 3142–3151.

12

STEM CELL CASE STUDIES, CHARTS & GRAPHS

CASE 1

Diagnosis: Osteoarthrosis (Gonarthrosis)

Age: 56 years/male

DESCRIPTION/TREATMENT:

Male patient, 56 years old, high performance athlete, begins with pain in both knees with predominance in left knee, progressive damage, in 2012 reports absolute limitation to practice any sport and even certain everyday activities became painful.

Autologous cell therapy obtained from minimally manipulated bone marrow stem cells was applied, which consisted of intrajoint injection, repeated three times, four months between each of them. Starting with the first application, persistent clinical improvement is detected, returning the patient to his daily activities without any limitation and permitting sports activities with intermittent minimal discomfort. On radiographic follow-up studies, we get evidence of absence of progression of joint deterioration in the last 2 years. Also, we can observe a larger space in the joint that could presuppose cartilage growth.

Due to the technical difficulties and implications of a comparative study, it is not always possible to reliably establish an improvement based on one image. It is suggested to corroborate results with an MRI and/or arthroscopic surgery.

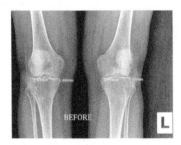 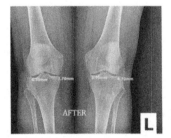

PATIENT COMMENTS:

"I used to exercise a lot. I used to play soccer and tennis and I did a lot of running. A few years ago, I was not able to perform these sports because it was too painful for my knees and after a workout my knees were swollen. Daily activities were also getting more and more painful, especially standing. A professional doctor, an "orthopedist", advised me to quit with these sports activities and focus on cycling. When the pain would get worse, the doctor would give me a knee replacement in the future. I didn't want to get a new knee, so I decided to do a stem cell treatment at ProgenCell. After three treatments my knees did not get weaker but stronger. I can stand still for a longer period of time painlessly in my day to day life. I also started running again and nowadays I can run 5 kilometers, practically with no pain" –JM

CASE 2

Diagnosis: Spinocerebellar Ataxia (SCA)

Age – 53/male

The patient is a basketball player and a health care professional. His problem began 5 years ago when it became increasingly difficult to play. Soon he developed intermittent diplopia (double vision) as well. He progressively also had problems with his balance, coordination, slurring of speech and excessive fatigue. Different neurologists gave varied diagnosis that was inconclusive and he was provisionally considered as a case of Spinocerebellar Ataxia .

REASON FOR COMING FOR TREATMENT:

The patient had tried all available conventional treatments in the best of neurology hospitals in several places even countries but there was no improvement. He then did his own research through various resources and decided to try new emerging treatments like stem cells, benefits of which he had heard about from other patients' groups suffering from similar disorders. There was level 5 evidence from peer reviewed medical journals on the efficacy of stem cells.

TREATMENT:

Mesenchymal Stem Cells derived from Wharton's Jelly of Human Umbilical cord. He received 6 injections of stem cells, 4 through Intravenous route in a dose of 1 million cells/kg body weight and 2 injections of adequate cells through intrathecal route.

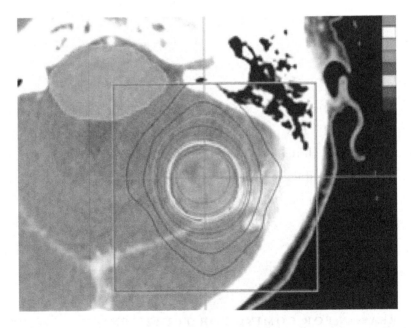

Before treatment: At the time of admission he was found to have following: Excessive fatigue, slurring of speech, lack of coordination, lack of balance.

After treatment: The following improvements were noticed by the medical team during the stay (just before discharge):

- There was a small improvement in his ability to perform coordinated movements. The finger nose test and heel to shin test also showed improvement.

- Tremors improved a little bit.

- He felt more energetic and in control of himself.

Further follow up is underway. Generally, improvements observed due to stem cells in most of the neurological diseases are limited if the primary disease is progressive in nature.

CASE 3:

Diagnosis: Multiple Sclerosis (MS)

Age: Male/59

Description of condition: The patient was unable to speak loud and clear. Muscular tension was increased on the left side. He felt "numb" in his left hand. Slight edema was noted in the left leg. Activity was limited in arms and legs. The alternate motion test was deemed "clumsy" in left arm. A shuffle was noted in his gait. Skin temperature was low in the legs. Skin color was blue, and it became worse when legs droop.

Treatment:

After admission, several medical protocols were applied, including:

- Treatment to improve neural function

- Promote cerebral blood circulation and metabolism, combined with Traditional Chinese Medicine (TCM) and rehabilitation therapy.

Physical Condition After Stem Cell Treatment for Multiple Sclerosis:

The patient's general condition improved significantly. He was able to speak with greater tone and volume. Muscle tension in left side improved. Numbness on the left hand diminished. The limbs became more flexible and muscle strength was improved. Walking and balance also improved. The shuffling gait disappeared. Skin temperature and skin color in lower limbs also improved, with a resolution of edema in the left leg.

CASE 4

Diagnosis: Chronic Obstructive Pulmonary Disease (COPD)

Age: 63 years/male

Source: ProgenCell Stem Therapies[4]

DESCRIPTION OF CONDITION:

A patient diagnosed with COPD (chronic obstructive pulmonary disease) due to high exposure to argon and asbestos in the construction and refinery industry. Allergic to sulfas without any additional health condition. At 55 years old started with bronchial symptoms. After being a smoker for 40+ years, quits smoking. The patient begins with a persistent cough, bronchial affectation and white-yellow phlegm progressing into a condition with respiratory distress. Studies confirm fibrosis and pleural thickening. Although the patient is actively independent, he has respiratory limitations that increase during physical activity.

TREATMENT:

Three treatments of autologous stem cell therapies at intervals of 4 and 10 months between them. Bone marrow aspiration was performed alternating both iliac crests selected as aspiration sites. After minimal lab processing, bone marrow is infused intravenously systemically. The following table shows the results of cell quantity and cell viability in each procedure:

Procedure	Date	Cell type & Source	Viability %	Mononuclear cell count	Infusion method
1st	Day 1	Hematopoietic cells – bone marrow	99.3	Total: 1500×10^6 Per ml: 750×10^4	IV
2nd	4 months	Hematopoietic cells – bone marrow	86.58	Total: 732×10^6 Per ml: 366×10^4	IV
3rd	14 months	Hematopoietic cells – bone marrow	97.28	Total: 3256×10^6 Per ml: 2713 $\times 10^3$	IV

EVOLUTION AFTER FIRST PROCEDURE:

The patient shows stable clinical conditions. No injury is shown in the aspiration site. Over a few months' patient reports no worsening of his symptoms and indicates no progression or discomfort. Shows improvement in breathing patterns and daily activities.

EVOLUTION AFTER SECOND PROCEDURE:

Patient shows stable clinical conditions. No bruise is shown on the aspiration site. During the following months patient shows improvement, increasing his capacity for daily activities and being able to walk with less fatigue.

Article: Administration of autologous bone marrow derived mononuclear cells in children with cerebral palsy[7]

SOURCE:

Sharma A, Gokulchandran N, Chopra G, Kulkarni P, Lohia M, Badhe P, V.C.Jacob. Administration of autologous bone marrow derived mononuclear cells in children with incurable neurological disorders and injury are safe and improves their quality of life. *Cell Transplantation*. 2012; 21 Supp 1: S1–S12.

Sharma et al, carried out a study on 71 children, wherein they administered 20 cases of cerebral palsy with autologous bone marrow mononuclear cells, intrathecally. These cases included dystonic and spastic CP. Symptoms commonly observed in them were delayed milestones, spasticity, motor impairment, ambulation deficits, cognitive impairment, swallowing and speech problems, etc. Autologous bone marrow MNCs were selected as they are easily obtainable, safe and do not involve any ethical issues. Intrathecal route of administration is a minimally invasive, safe and an effective procedure as compared to other routes. Studies[3][5][6] have also proved that a mixture of cells exhibits more benefits as compared to a single sub fraction of cells. Hence, intrathecal autologous BMMNC transplantation was carried out.

The patients were administered with Granulocyte Colony Stimulating Factor (GCSF), 48 hours and 24 hours before the harvest and transplantation of BMMNC. On the day of the transplantation, bone marrow was aspirated under general anesthesia in the operating theatre with aseptic precautions. Approximately, 100 ml of bone marrow (varying between 80 ml and 100 ml, based on the age and body weight) were aspirated from the region of anterior superior iliac spine using the bone marrow aspiration needle and collected in the heparinized tubes.

The aspirate was then transferred to the laboratory where the mononuclear cells were separated by the density gradient method. CD34+ counting was done by fluorescence-activated cell sorting (FACS). The MNCs were checked for viability (Average viability count was found to be 97%).

The separated autologous BMMNCs were immediately injected on the same day, intrathecally using an 18G Touhy needle and an epidural catheter at the level between fourth and fifth lumbar vertebrae. Simultaneously 20mg/kg body weight methyl prednisolone in 500 ml Ringer Lactate was given intravenously to enhance survival of the injected cells. The patient was monitored for any adverse events.

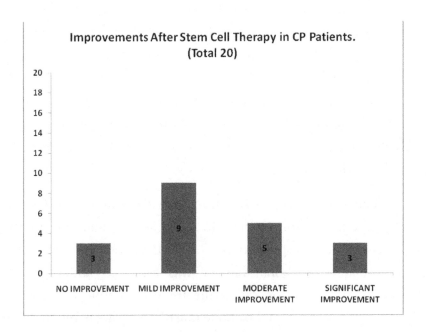

On mean follow up of 15-months $\pm$ 1-month post stem cell administration, improvement was observed in 85% cases. Significant improvement was observed in spasticity, neck holding, drooling of saliva, muscle strength in upper and lower limbs, sitting and standing balance, gross and fine motor activities, speech, swallowing, ambulation, and cognition. There was also a reduction in dystonic movements. No major adverse events were recorded. Some minor side effects such as headache, nausea, and vomiting were experienced by few children who were self-limiting (resolved within a week) and treated with medications. The improvements in these patients sustained even after the follow up period of the study. None of them showed any deterioration on the GMFCS.

OTHER CASES: FANCONI'S ANEMIA

Molly Nash's story gives a clear illustration as to how stem cell therapy can improve and save lives. Molly had Fanconi's anemia, a genetic blood disease. People who suffer such ailments do not live until adulthood. They die in infancy or early teenage age. A bone marrow transplant from a healthy sibling with a matched HLA or immune profile can cure the disease, but Molly was an only child and her parents — both carriers of the deadly gene — were fearful of having another child with the disease. They used in vitro fertilization, pre-implantation diagnosis (PGD) and a cord blood transplant in an attempt to save their child. PGD was used to screen 24 embryos made in the laboratory. One embryo was disease-free and matched Molly's immune profile. The blastocyst was implanted and nine months later her sibling, named Adam, was born. The stem cells from Adam's umbilical cord were given to Molly and today she is eleven years old and free from disease.

REFERENCES

1.   Bone Marrow Transplantation and Peripheral Blood Stem Cell Transplantation in National Cancer Institute Fact Sheet web site. Bethesda, MD: National Institutes of Health, U.S. Department of Health and Human Services, 2010. Cited 24 August 2010.

2.   Karanes C, Nelson GO, Chitphakdithai P, Agura E, Ballen KK, Bolan CD, Porter DL, Uberti JP, King RJ, Confer DL (2008). "Twenty years of unrelated donor hematopoietic cell transplantation for adult recipients facilitated by the National Marrow Donor Program." *Biology of Blood and Marrow Transplantation.* **14** (9 Suppl): 8-15. PMID 18721775

3.   Malard F, Mohty M (2014). "New Insight for the Diagnosis of Gastrointestinal Acute Graft- versus- host Disease." *Meditators Inflamm.* 2014: 701013. PMC 3964897. PMID 24733964

4.   Teixeira, Fabio G; Carvalho, Miguel M; Sousa, Nuno; Salgado, Antonio J (2013). "Mesenchymal Stem Cells Secretome: a new paradigm for central for central nervous system regeneration?" *Cellular and Molecular Life Sciences.* **70** (20): 3871-3882. ISSN 1420-682X

5.   Rosemann A (2014). "Why regenerative stem cell medicine progresses slower than expected." *J Cell Biochem.* **115** (12): 2073-76. PMID 25079695

6.   Maguire, G (2016). "Therapeutics from Adult Stem Cells and the Hype Curve." *ACS Medicinal Chemistry Letter.* **7** (5): 441-43. PMID 27190588

7.   Sharma A, Gokulchandran N, Chopra G, Kulkarni P, Lohia M, Badhe P, V.C.Jacob. Administration of autologous bone marrow derived mononuclear cells in children with incurable neurological disorders and injury is safe and improves their quality of life. Cell Transplantation. 2012; 21 Supp 1: S1–S12.

8.   Christopher Scott. STEM CELL NOW. PI Press (Penguin books) 2006.

13

THE FUTURE OF
STEM CELLS

Healthcare statistics are very scary. Over 2 million Americans are projected to contract End Stage Renal Disease, with a whooping cost of about $1 trillion to the state. One therefore wonders what role modern medicine will play to alleviate such suffering. In 2001, more than 80,000 patients required organ transplants. Of these, fewer than 24,000 people got them. 6,000 died in the process of waiting. 40 percent of those who successfully got the transplant died three years after the surgery. One in five of our elders (65 years old or older) will require temporary or permanent organ repair or replacement during their remaining years. In 2002, the prevalence of diabetes in the United States exceeded 18 million people — 6.3 percent of the population. That year, total healthcare costs of diabetes surpassed $130 billion. More than 1,500 people are killed by cancer daily.

As we can see there are problems to be solved; the greater

the problem, the harder the solution to it. The more people you can help solving the problem, the is more money involved in such problem. Therefore many groups are investing lots of resources in research in order to solve those problems, and Stem Cell research has shown promise to be part of the solution. We can be sure this subject will not be forgotten in a few years, it will become a very important branch of the practice of medicine. Stem Cell technology can be clearly described as a revolution in research. Unlocking the hidden potential of cells to help repair and rebuild the human body is indeed a revolution.

Nobody can predict the future, of course, but it is easy to perceive two main paths of stem cell therapy development: Treatment for the masses and individual treatments.

TREATMENT FOR THE MASSES

In short, this path is about treating Stem Cells as a drug. The goal is to have a product or series of products on hospital and pharmacies shelves, available to treat great groups of people. Even though this path is easy to summarize in a few lines, it is actually a complicated multifactor subject. We will try to give you the idea in the following paragraphs.

In order to develop technology, resources have to be invested. The more complicated the problem to solve, the more research there needs to be done and therefore more resources are implicated. Who has the resources to invest in medical technology and have some kind of interest?

It is hard to see how the future will develop, but it seems like pharmaceutical companies are investing a lot of money to research on stem cells, everyone wants to be part of it. And they are a very important piece of the puzzle when it comes to developing new drugs, medical instruments, etc.

What kind of research will they invest on? The financially beneficial, and that is the one where your market is a large group of people with a similar disease. Large corporations focus on Diabetes, Rheumatoid Arthritis, Parkinson's, Cancer, etc. While rare diseases with less patients are left behind.

It is expected that the pharmaceutical industry will develop products to sell for the masses, while smaller groups and independent medical practices develop services for orphan diseases. Private investment from smaller groups will be needed to develop a bedside treatment taking advantage of the full power of stem cells.

From our point of view, it is a huge challenge for pharmaceutical companies to create a product like a "drug": one size fits most, which you could find at any pharmacy. There are many factors to solve before we can see it possible.

A strategy to reduce cost. Instead of creating a unique Stem Cell line for each individual, it could be much better to create and develop several thousand banks of HESC lines. Each line could then be tested by means of a histocompatibility antigen typing procedure (HLA). This would drastically minimize the chances of tissue rejection. The closer the HLA match (either from family members or from outside donors), the less the chance that rejection will be a problem. A similar list of donors already exists. Over 6.5 million individuals have already been HLA-typed for bone marrow registries.

WHEN?

Stem cell holds a lot of promise, especially in regards of the replacement of body parts lost to injury, aging, wear and tear, and even infirmity. However, the unfortunate thing is that the reality of Stem Cell therapy is overhyped. For instance, it is believed that in the future, everyone will have an unlimited access to Stem Cells, just walk into the hospital and you will have it in whatever quantity you need. Such hype!

What do you need? A new pancreas? New cardiac tissue? You want to grow some new villi in your intestine? There's something for you! That's how far the hype has gone. Thus, patients of the 21st century may get to believe that they can prolong their lives with some medical patchwork.

This may sound like an exciting future. But it will take time — and vision — to us get there.

The truth of the matter is; we've got a good distance to go before regenerative medicine — a catchall term for Stem Cell therapy — will help large numbers of patients. It is very possible that many diseases will have to wait for cures from other quarters of medicine. Before any medical treatment (including cell and tissue transplants) is made available through hospitals or clinics, it must first be tested in humans through tightly regulated phases of clinical trials. The first phase determines safety and side effects in a few dozen subjects; the second phase tests the efficacy in hundreds of patients; the third and subsequent phases try to prove statistical significance and confirm its effects in many hundreds or thousands of patients. The U.S. Food and Drug Administration (FDA) evaluate the data, and if the results pass muster, the product is approved for sale and moves in the market.

It is very tedious and quite difficult to develop a new therapy, much worse is the expenses involved in developing one. You'll have to conduct a research, make a discovery, test, and perform clinical trials. This would cost not less than a billion dollars and would take about 10 – 15 years to realize[2].

An estimated duration for modern skin transplants may have an outline similar to the one below:

- **Basic Research:** 2006 marks the discovery of very potent adult Stem Cells lying underneath the human skin. These cells, which are extremely rare, are fingerprinted by genetic markers and then isolated for culturing in the laboratory. Over the next two years, technology is developing to grow the cells in quantity and used to change them into a variety of skin cell types.

- **Preclinical Research:** A transgenic mouse with no immune system was selected to prevent rejection of the human cells. Different lines of Stem Cells from skin, along with their progenitors, are transplanted into the mouse's injured skin. Over time the transplants are observed. One-line works: the cells survive, go to the site of the injury, integrate into the skin, and heal the wound. Other kinds of animals are similarly tested. The tests take three years to complete.

Clinical Research: The encouraging results in animals' prompt tests in humans. In cases of patients with severe burns, stem cells of their own skin are cultured, multiplied and then transplanted at the wound site. The cells improve blood flow, promote healing, and reduce scarring. Using adult Stem Cells is not the only way to approach the problem. The technologies are further developed by companies, tested in more humans, and manufactured for use for burn victims. In 2014, the FDA approves the first cell therapy for use in clinics [4].

If the treatment being studied is for a disease with a genetic cause, another wrinkle must be ironed out. Before the transplant could succumb with time or the cells are reintroduced, the faulty gene has to be corrected. This poses a new set of problems to Stem Cell transplants. If a modified Stem Cell is grated into a body tissue or organ, it may remain there for life. If the modification takes place in one of the most mobile elements of the human body, such as the blood cells, then you can be sure that in no time, every part of the body will record the change. Therefore, it is best to take precautionary measures before delving into such.

Some experts contend that individual treatments are feasible, and that once the competition heats up, market forces will conspire to bring down prices. They argue that if Stem cell therapy can cure, then all the downstream costs of caring for chronic illness go away. An initially high price for injecting Stem Cells would be more than offset by future medical savings.

However, even with the concerns of time and money, there is plenty of good news. Stem Cells are already used in clinics with resounding success.

STEM CELLS AS TOOLS

The Experts agree that immortal embryonic lines will become one of biology's most powerful tools. A pioneer of in vitro fertilization, Alan Trounson, an Australian stem cell biologist and embryologist, believes that "studying disease with Stem Cells is incredibly important for research. We need to develop embryonic cell lines from patients who've got Muscular Dystrophy, Alzheimer's disease, and Cystic Fibrosis. That way we can develop drugs that actually block the disease from occurring.". James Thomson agrees. "Human embryonic Stem Cell research will be developed more as a research tool than for transplanting engineered cells and tissues. I mean, think about disease for a minute," he says. "You don't want to do anything so crude as replacing those cells once they have died. You want to stop the disease from happening in the first place! If you had a reliable supply of neuronal cells, for example, you could study them to understand exactly how Alzheimer's disease causes them to die."

Discovering drug is an important application of HESC technology. Drugs to be used in the treatment of a particular disease could be tested in a population of cells that have been affected by that disease. A classic example would be the case of neurons that produce dopamine in a state of Parkinson's Disease. Such neurons could be derived from HESC lines and preserved in large amounts.

Treating the neurons and measuring their response would quickly sort out which chemicals work best. Thousands of potential drugs tested in this fashion would speed up drug discovery. Existing pharmaceuticals could be refined and improved in the same fashion.

Gene therapy is a relatively recent and highly experimental approach to treating diseases. Although most drugs are manufactured outside the body, gene therapy takes a different approach: a gene is delivered into the affected cells in the body, where it produces a protein that acts as a therapeutic agent. The potential success depends not only on the gene delivery into the appropriate cells, but also on the gene's ability to function properly. Both requirements pose considerable technical challenges. Noninfectious viruses are used to deliver the gene, just like ordinary viruses infect cells. Unfortunately, this method is imprecise and also limited to the specific types of cells the virus can infect. If the proteins aren't produced efficiently or the transformed cells eventually die of old age, then repeated rounds of therapy are needed.

Gene therapy can be improved by using Stem Cells. Because Stem Cells self-renew, they can reduce the need for repeated rounds of therapy. Blood-forming Stem Cells are easily removed from — and reintroduced into — the body, and after getting into the body the hone in on different organs like thymus, spleen, and marrow. Thus, they are good choices for delivering drugs. Dozens of human clinical trials have used HSCs to deliver therapeutic agents such as interferon to patients suffering from blood and solid-tumor cancers (as opposed to cancers of the blood), anemias, and immune diseases such as SCID and HIV. In some cases, the results have been promising, extending the lives of terminally ill patients. Another way to deliver a therapeutic gene is cell-to-cell fusion, a phenomenon behind apparent Stem Cell plasticity. If the disease is due to a missing or defective gene in the liver, an engineered blood stem cell might fuse with liver cells and produce the needed protein. Though, fusion is a rare event, so it may be a problem to deliver enough protein for repairing the organ[1].

Neuroscientist Anders Bjorklun believes that combining genes with Stem Cell therapy could hold the solution to brain damage/

dysfunction. Delivering a corrected copy of Nurr1 to patients through Stem Cells could impede the progression of Parkinson's disease. The thought here is to insert a perfect corrected copy of the gene into a virgin cell. A lot of such genetically modified cells could be injected into the brain. If the cells took hold, they would manufacture the missing protein. Bjorklund adds that cells that promote brain healing and self-repair could be injected. The big hurdle here is navigating the pathways of cell differentiation. According to Bjorkund, "One of our dilemmas is that we don't always know what is, and what is not a nervous system Stem Cell."

Experiments using other kinds of Stem Cells to carry therapeutic cargo are underway. High-powered mesenchymal cells carrying the cancer-fighting gene for interferon doubled the survival rates in transgenic mice ridden with human tumors. The cells honed in on tumors no matter their location, suggesting a way to treat human cancers that have already spread. Stem Cells of the nervous system, which carry anti-tumor agents such as Interleukin-2, are also promising.

Experiments carried out in mice with brain tumors show that the Stem Cells synthesize and secrete interleukin-2, which then triggers chemotaxis and phagocytosis by the white blood cells. Other Stem Cells could deliver the drugs to the target with 100 percent precision.

Stem Cells are being used to diagnose diseases. At a growing number of in vitro fertilization clinics, single-gene defects that cause Huntington's, Tay Sachs, Sickle Cell Anemia, Cystic Fibrosis, and dozens of other disorders are being detected via an embryo-sampling technique called preimplantation genetic diagnosis, or PGD. Four days after fertilization, while still in a laboratory dish, an eight-cell embryo is grasped gently by light suction and a single cell is removed with a pipette. The embryo recovers with a quick round of cell division. The DNA in the cell is extracted and then tested with a genetic probe for the disease in question. The tests give a clue as to whether the embryo is a disease carrier or not. Embryos without the disease gene will implanted, while those with the disease gene will be discarded. Parents who carry the gene, or who have family histories of the disease, can use PGD to avoid having an affected child. A separate analysis identifies a group of different disorders caused by the wrong chromosome number, such as Down's syndrome, or abnormalities that lead to miscarriage. PGD has emerged as a tool for parents whose only other option would be to test abnormalities during fetal development. In most cases, PGD enables the family to avoid the difficult decision of whether or not to end a late stage pregnancy. The procedure is expensive, running $5,000 for both sets of tests.

Just as advances in reproductive biology helped embryologists derive the first human embryonic Stem Cell lines, PGD can help study diseases. Instead of doing away with infected and disease-laden embryos, a research institute in Chicago has developed 30 HESC lines and used them as research materials. Researchers can now use them as in vitro models. Observing how these cells behave compared to normal cells will help identify how certain diseases begin, progress, and affect healthy tissue. Not only are the disease-causing genes and their proteins identified, this also opens up possibilities for designing drugs that reverse or treat the problem [3].

The diversity of Stem Cell treatments reflects the diversity of Stem Cell breeds. Lines of HESCs may become a standardize source of cells used to treat patients. At the moment, bone marrow and tissue engineering together with early clinical trials have verified the viability of adult Stem Cells. Both kinds of cells could take different paths, their differences here need further research.

INDIVIDUAL TREATMENTS

This path is about practice of medicine, using Stem Cells from the same patient (autologous) and sometimes using Stem Cells from other sources. It would be a relationship between the caregiver and the patient; it is not about a product to use, is about taking care of the patient, and customizing the different therapies available to the patient needs. If the patient has a knee problem Stem Cell therapy will be very different than a patient with an degenerative autoimmune disease. It cannot be treated with the same pill, in the same dose. Different lab process will be used to prepare the cells.

By now most of the properties of Stem Cells are known, finding a better way to take advantage of the full potential that Stem Cells have is the challenge. In the future some technologies will evolve finding a better way to:

- Improve the technique of Stem Cell release/placement in the body.

- Create a proper environment in the body for the cells to engraft and perform better, by using alternative therapies and substances.

- Concentrate the cells into specific organs and transport the cells into specific places. Placement of the cells will be more specific, For example, the use of nanotechnology, viral transportation, attachment to magnetic particles and then electromagnetism to guide them. All these will help concentrate the cells in the tissue to be repaired.

- Better stimulation for the cells to become active and keep active for the long run. Increasing activity related to regenerative power, avoiding just cell blending or being immune-unidentified and discarded.

- Use growth factors to stimulate cell differentiation into specific tissues.

- Use of peptides, enzymes or other molecules.

- Produce scaffolds, right now there are 3D printers making scaffolds to help Stem Cells engraft and duplicate, but those scaffolds are not good enough to replicate an actual organ. Once we are able to replicate them and make it fully functional, then we will be challenged on how to introduce or replace the current tissue structure without making damage to surrounding structures. Then another challenge will emerge, since the body is a growing mechanism, a static scaffold won't be enough, dynamic scaffolds that grow into the body and the body integrates as its own will be developed.

With all these happening the health improvements that the patients will get will be better and last longer.

To increase efficiency on the cell behavior there are two main factors: Genetic information and the surrounding environment. When both of them sync on the positive side, the cells work and behave better. Research of how to improve the genetic information and how to improve the microenvironment of the cells is crucial for better outcomes. Understanding and combining the use of hormone therapy, enzymes, surrounding nutrition of the cells, among others will become key for every medical practice.

As more knowledge on the genetic field becomes available and gene editing with technologies such as CRISPR; Stem Cells will be able to be directed to specific tissues, and differentiate into specific cells. Since genetic information is unique for each person, autologous Stem Cells could be manipulated with that genetic information of that specific patient to grow his specific tissue or specific differentiated cell to be implanted only in his body. This could be the road to create structures/tissues of different organs, without being genetically specific, for example using allogenic or IPSC, there is a big probability of engraftment and function failure.

HOW MUCH?

Customized treatments that can't rely on economics of scale are likely to be very expensive. For an adult Stem Cell regime, the tissue in which the Stem Cells reside must be biopsied — perhaps more than once. For any cell therapy the methods for isolating, growing, and expanding the cultures must be perfected. The procedure must give rise to an unlimited number of Stem Cells, which must have a long-life span. Also, it must be unique, pure and free of contaminants such as bacteria, viruses and other pathogens.

We already know how to collect Stem Cells, process them, cryo-preserve them, and infuse them for some degenerative diseases, but there is a long road to the full effect expected from this type of cells. We will discover in the future the middle steps that need to be taken in order learn how to release the cells in the right place, with the right growth factors and the right dose.

REGULATION

Since there is a lot of potential behind the subject of Stem Cell therapy, some people will take advantage of patients with health crisis. Local regulation is very important to mitigate non-professionals that sell "cures" to anyone willing to pay.

Nowadays we have a problem where many families expect too much from Stem Cells, and the hype is so big that many even expect a miracle for their family member. You might hear that Stem Cell therapy does not work just because it did not meet the miracle expected, even if there were some minor improvements. Maybe some of this deception also comes from creating false expectations from the current non-professional providers.

Governments are developing legislations to prevent those non-professionals from taking advantage of patients who are not so well informed. Regulation is getting tougher. Every month clinics, hospitals, and doctors who will be willing to follow guidelines and quality control will have a hard time to comply, but in the long run is really beneficial for patients. Today you can even see a quick multiplication of health providers happening, many medical and esthetical offices are or will be adding to their services Stem Cell therapy, but after a few months or even a few years those providers that do not comply with the guidelines of the FDA, COFEPRIS or whichever health authority they have in their location, will rapidly disappear.

VACCINES

Another change in the near future to expect is related to vaccines.

Vaccines are very important to eradicate very important diseases. Most pediatricians recommend them because they have proven to protect children and to prevent an outbreak and spread dangerous virus. But on the other hand, vaccines are basically toxic to the body. There are studies that prove that injecting a low diminished virus can trigger devastating effects in the body such as autism in children.

As time goes by, you can expect a change of practice where vaccines are going to be used only when the immunologic system is not strong enough or is compromised. Therefore, vaccines would be used only in groups and geographical areas where they are needed: such as rural areas without proper hygene, without good nutrition, without good resources or in places where there are still cases of this type of active virus. The practice to vaccine ALL babies being born will disappear someday. There is another problem, but that is not related to health, is related to financial interest: How much money is involved behind the vaccine industry.

We would like to see a future with selective vaccination and more preventive treatments reinforcing the immune system such as Stem Cell therapy.

CONCLUSION

It is becoming more common to see people over 100 yrs old. In the future it will start to be common to see people over 120 yrs old. This does not mean that people 120 yrs old will be healthy; it means that people with 100 yrs old will have a good condition to enjoy life and be able to get older than today.

In the near future, patients will have more knowledge about Stem Cell therapy and caregivers will manage expectations more realistically. This type of therapy will find its place, it will become the gold standard for some diseases, pricing will also be adjusted, and insurance will start to cover this kind of expense. Stem Cells will not be a cure for everything. Anti-aging treatments will become a frequent protocol. The number of medical conditions that today are being marketed as treatable with Stem Cells, will be reduce to a few, and of course, other uses for Stem Cells will be discovered.

The goal should be to get our body into a better condition, by doing so it will last longer. The healthier you are, the fewer drugs and treatments you need. Today people are healthier because of hygene awareness, better physical activity habits and better nutrition. Good habits will reflect automatically in your body as a strong immune system, requiring less medical care (of course there are exceptions on medical conditions triggered by external factors or even gene information).

We encourage our readers to invest time and money in their health by creating the microenvironment in their body to let the perfection of the human body to work its natural healing and regenerative functions. Invest with continuous dedication to be physically active, spiritually/mentally balanced and with a healthy diet. If your specific case needs some extra help, then let's discuss Stem Cell therapy.

REFERENCES

1. Anne McLaren Laboratory for Regenerative Medicine: Stem Cells: The Future of Medicine?"

2. EuroStemCell: iPS cells and reprogramming: turn any cell of the body into a stem cell," Sept. 15, 2015

3. Minerva Biotechnologica: "Adult-derived stem cells,", Vol. 17, No. 2:55-63 (2005)

4. Totipotent Stem Cells are present in the Blood of Adult Equines," Keystone Symposium (2007)

5. Method of Stimulating and Extracting Non-embryonic Pluripotent Cells from Mammal Blood and Using Reconstituted Pluripotent Cells to Treat Disease Including Chronic Obstructive Pulmonary Disease," Royal et al., USPTO Application Number 13362993 (2011)

14

A GUIDE ON HOW TO FIND THE RIGHT STEM CELL TREATMENT CLINIC

Stem Cell Treatment has enormous potential to help scientist and doctors treat and get a better understanding a wide range of injuries and diseases. For over 30 years, bone marrow (because of its high concentration of Stem Cells) has been used to treat cancer patients with conditions such as leukemia and lymphoma. During chemotherapy, most growing cells are killed by the cytotoxic agents. These agents, however, cannot discriminate between the leukaemia or neoplastic cells, and the hematopoietic stem cells within the bone marrow. It is this side effect of conventional chemotherapy strategies that the stem-cell transplant attempts to reverse; a donor's healthy bone marrow reintroduces functional stem cells to replace the cells lost in the host's body during treatment.

But, it is also important to understand that we still have a lot to learn about Stem Cells and their therapeutic use. Unfortunately, stem Cell treatment is commonly approached in a negative way by the media, and most of the time they don't really understand the science behind it, and also by doctors looking to make an unethical profit, by selling treatments to chronically ill or seriously injured patients. What we will try cover in this chapter, is to provide you with the basic understanding of Stem Cell Treatments, it's potential, and it's limitations. And also, a reference to prevent you from falling into the arms of a fraudster.

What You Should Know Before Considering Stem Cell Treatment

There is certain information you should know before considering stem cell treatment, especially when considering an option outside your country. We have compiled a list of five things to consider, even before searching for a Stem Cell treatment center.

STEM CELL TREATMENT IS NOT A MIRACLE CURE FOR EVERY DISEASE AND IS NOT FOR EVERYONE.

Stem Cell Treatment is not a cure. If someone is advertising or proposing Stem Cell treatment as a cure for a Chronic Diseases, they are lying. There are some diseases and injuries on which stem cell treatment has been proven to be beneficial. But it is not a miracle cure.

A STEM CELL TREATMENT MUST COMPLY WITH
REGULATIONS, REGARDLESS OF THE COUNTRY.

Stem cell therapies are regulated differently in various countries around the world, with some countries offering stem cell therapies that are not available elsewhere.

These differences depend entirely on the government policy of each country. But, this does not mean that a stem cell treatment outside your country must not comply with regulations. For example, in Mexico, all doctors, clinics and hospitals are regulated by COFEPRIS (the Mexican version of the FDA) a federal agency, that regulates all health services providers in Mexico. Countries like Mexico enjoy a substantial economic benefit from medical tourism, and the government is constantly working on ensuring that medical providers offer a top quality and safe medical services.

Stem Cell Treatment Potential & Limitations

Cell therapy is not a solution to all existing health problems. Each person reacts differently; the main purpose of this procedure is to give tools to the body and create ideal conditions to generate damaged tissue by itself. Past experiences and procedures show a great improvement in the majority of patients while other patients may not show substantial improvement.

How to Search for Stem Cell Treatment Center

If you are considering Stem Cell Treatment as an alternative to improve your quality of life, or regain control of your life. The first thing to figure out is to how to search for the right Stem

Cell Treatment Clinic, the best suitable for your condition, your family and your budget.

Having your loved ones involved in the decision. A decision like undergoing a stem cell treatment has to be considered and measured surrounded by friends and family that can help you along the path, and can also input with a much wider perspective. When dealing with a difficult to bear medical condition, the hope for a cure can obnubilate our judgement and make us take a wrong decision, with undesirable consequences.

Medical Tourism is currently an alternative to seek medical treatments outside your country at affordable prices. Stem Cell Treatment can also fall in the category of circumvention tourism, which is to travel in order to access medical services that are regulated in the destination country but not regulated in the home country. The first place to go when searching for Medical Tourism is the internet. When looking for a Stem Cell Treatment Center on the internet, you shouldn't always trust the Center or the doctors website and/or social media profiles. Remember that the website, and it's content, is created and moderated by the doctor or clinic itself. Becoming judge and a party at the same time. What you should look in to, is the reputation of the center in a third party website. Make sure that the ratings, are coming from sources were the center or doctor cannot edit or manipulate. And also, to be fair, always check into the doctor reply.

If you are not the kind of person that likes "Do it yourself" projects, you can seek help from a professional medical planner. This is very important when considering Stem Cell Treatment abroad. There are medical tourism facilitators and patient advocate services that can help you find the right service for you and can become an important ally when searching for Stem Cell Treatment Center, abroad.

What to Ask When Considering Stem Cell Therapy:

WHAT ARE THE CLINIC CREDENTIALS?

Regardless of the country you are looking at for Stem Cell Treatments, the Clinic or Stem Cell Treatment has to comply with regulations. You need to ask for the local regulations, and make sure that the doctors have proper and updated local credentials.

IS THE TREATMENT IN A HOSPITAL OR AN SPECIALIZED STEM CELL TREATMENT CENTER?

Stem Cell Treatment is a relatively new kind of treatment. Some doctors have trained online quickly or taken a 2 hr crash course and they feel ready to offer Stem Cell Treatment in their office or the Hospital where they commonly work. It is risky to go to a doctor who has another specialty and as a bonus he/she does stem cells injections. You should consider a clinic that is specifically designed for Stem Cell Treatment, preferably with an adjacent stem cell laboratory and right equipment (medical and scientifically) .

HOW MUCH EXPERIENCE YOUR DOCTORS HAVE?

Even though Stem Cell Treatment is relatively new, this doesn't mean that doctors shouldn't have several years of experience. Stem Cell Treatment has been done for over 30 years, and doctors performing it should have several years of experience and the proper training.

WHAT CELL SOURCE ARE YOU USING?

A Stem Cell Treatment should assertively answer this question every time. You need to know what is the source of the Stem Cells being used and whether it is an allogeneic or an autologous treatment. If the clinic does not tell you where does the stem cells come from, that means they are hiding something. Maybe there is something wrong, You should know if the stem cells are yours, from a 3rd party, animal cell, or plant cells. You have to feel comfortable about where they come from, what quality assurance process will they go through before infusion. Skipping this step increases your risk enormously.

HOW DO YOU MAKE SURE THE STEM CELLS ARE PLACED WHERE THEY'RE NEEDED MOST?

This is a very important question and the answer is not obvious, as it may seem. You need to look for a Stem Cell delivery method not only effective, but also safe. When dealing with a heart disease, the safest way is not to inject directly into the heart. The safest approach is to deliver the Stem Cells intravenously; this way is safer and equally effective.

WHAT IS THE CLINIC SUCCESS RATE AND HOW DO YOU MEASURE SUCCESS?

Success is totally relative to expectation. Consider 2 different athletes who have succeeded they succeed running a mile. They both can tell you they had 100% success, but to you it may seem different when you find out that one of them ran the mile in 8 min while the other ran it barely in 30 min. We tend to believe that numbers offer an accurate measurement of things. But this is not always the case, is of highly importance to understand what is being measured and how is being measured. Success rate is the average of patients with successful outcomes (related to expectations), what is interesting or important to us, is to truly comprehend what the doctor considers a successful outcome. It only works when the expectations of the doctor and of the patient are aligned. Even the most careful physicians have patients who develop complications depending on the current condition of the patient. Unfortunately, in the field of medicine, these things happen. Physicians or clinics that tell you they have a 100% success rate or close are lying, manipulating their numbers, or have their expectations really low. It would be nice to have access those patients and ask them if their case was successful, then we will be able to align expectations of the doctor and the patient. Ask your doctor what his success rate is, and then what he considers success for the stem cell procedure you're considering. If the doctor 's answer includes a realistic view of success and failure, then you have a physician who is being honest.

WHAT WILL THE COST BE?

Every clinic or doctor you are considering for Stem Cell Treatment should be very clear about what costs you will incur, including costs of a complication or an emergency. Ask about traveling expenses, lodging, airfare, medications, and/or medical fees. If it's a clinical trial, ask if it's patient funded or if the cost of treatment and trial monitoring is covered by the company developing the product or by local or national government funding.

Before making the decision, you need to know exactly what costs you will or may incur. This information is not only financially wise, it will also mean your doctor or clinic have thoroughly reviewed your case.

What You Should Know Before Making Your Decision

ABOUT THE TREATMENT

Before deciding whether or not Stem Cell treatment is the route to take, you need to make sure that you understand your expectation related to the Stem Cell treatment.

You need to make sure that the treatment is developed for your specific disease or condition being treated, make sure the sources of the cells, call the doctor and make sure he will be able to talk to you in case you need to contact him after the procedure, make sure they have the proper facilities and the proper equipment, ask if the treatment is part of a formal clinical trial.   Answering the questions of what? who? where? how? Will give you a complete perspective in order to make a right decision.

It's important that you know what are the alternative options to treat your disease or condition. Also, make sure that the Stem Cell Treatment does not interfere with any other medical treatment.

The treatment plan should be concise and precise on what are the possible benefits you can expect, how will this benefits be measured and how long will this take. What other medications or special care you might need. How will the stem cell procedure be done:

- What is the source of the stem cells?

- How are the stem cells identified, isolated and grown?

- Are the cells differentiated into specialized cells before therapy?

- How are the cells delivered to the right part of the body?

- If the cells are not my own, how will my immune system be prevented from reacting to the transplanted cells?

SCIENTIFIC EVIDENCE

Science should be consistent with the Stem Cell procedure. Make sure to read and learn as much as you can about Stem Cells and their nature. You need to know what is the scientific evidence that this procedure will work. How many clinical trials have been performed before the treatment, and what scientific conclusions have been drawn from these trials. Whenever you hear there are patients rejected from one kind of treatment, you have assurance that they are not there for the business side of the person, they are interested on the medical side of the patient.

Every new treatment should have an oversight by an ethics committee.

SAFETY AND EMERGENCIES

Every Stem Cell Treatment provider should make aware of the risks of the procedure itself, and the possible side effects both immediate and long-term. Regardless of how simple a medical procedure, has risks and reported side effects. Every Stem Cell

Clinic should be adequately prepared to handle emergencies such as a serious allergic reaction. A comprehensive treatment follow up should be provided by the clinic, and specific about how long these follow up treatment is. A doctor has to bee in charge in every part of the procedure, you should know who this doctor is, and how to communicate with him or her.

PATIENT RIGHTS

You have the right to be informed of any new information that might come up. You also have the right to withdraw from the treatment process at anytime. You should be guaranteed access to information, fair treatment, and autonomy over medical decisions, among other rights. You need to make sure, to understand and know your rights as patient. Beware of guaranteed medical treatments. No doctor can guarantee any kind of result of any kind of medical treatment; the only thing that can be guaranteed is that you are receiving a proper medical treatment by a licensed physician.

Warning Signs:

- **A CURE**

  You should be very careful with clinic offering Stem Cell Treatments as magical cures.

- **UNREGULATED CLINICS**

  Every clinic or doctor should be able to present their credentials. Beware of unregulated Stem Cell Treatment Centers (even in the US).

- **SUCCESS RATE**

  Beware of physicians or clinics that tell you they have a 100% success rate or close to it.

- **GUARANTEED RESULTS**

  In medicine, there is no way to guarantee results. Even the most careful and prepared physician cannot guarantee a result.

15

THE IMPORTANCE OF GOOD NUTRITION FOR STEM CELL THERAPY

A good and balanced diet is an essential part of a healthy lifestyle. The choices of food can largely affect an individual's body at a cell level reflected on overall health and wellbeing. A healthy diet can be the essential key in having a positive outlook in life and become emotionally balanced individual. Healthy food eating habits can help your cells live longer, replenish your organs to operate more efficiently, the mind and feel better. If a person's food choices are very unhealthy, a negative impact in the body is expected to happen.

People having unhealthy eating habits create a harmful microenvironment at a cell level promoting cell damage therefore they are subject to acquire diseases such as diabetes, different heart problems, stroke, hypertension, obesity and some certain types of cancer. Nobody wants to get sick and have a dreaded disease with unknown cure. However, you can prevent this from happening if you start a habit of eating healthy with added physical activities that can boost your metabolism for an effective way of maintaining a healthier weight.

Engaging to different exercises and physical activities can improve your wellness and make this as an important part of your healthy lifestyle. It provides many health benefits needed by an elder adult to stay physically active as well as the young adult ones. A regular, moderate exercise activity can help improve physical health of frail individuals and elders with diseases related to aging. Exercising can actually help an individual look more youthful and glowing. Strenuous activities for the elders can be challenging but there are a lot of good reasons why you have to do this and get moving. No matter what age or present state an individual may have, be as proactive as possible as this can produce long term health benefits.

Stem cells travel through different tissues and become the working cells of a certain vital organ in the body. It can tremendously help and treat different ranges of diseases, injuries and other health-related conditions. These cells have a remarkable potential to differentiate into many different types of cell as it also serves as an internal repair system, dividing essentially without limit as it continuously renewing themselves through cell division. Inside a healthy body, these stem cells have the capability to replicate many times for longer periods compared to your muscle cells and nerve cells. A combination of a healthy diet and regular exercise will lead to a healthier body. Having the proper microenvironment surrounding the stem cells, lead to a better engraftment, easier for them to duplicate and ultimately differentiate to repair tissue and replace inefficient cells. Therefore, a healthy lifestyle is key to get the most benefits out of the power of stem cells.

GENERAL GOOD EATING HABITS

Human nutritional needs differ with each life age stages. In order to stay healthy, it's important to take into consideration these nutritional demands with each age stage.

Generally, you can meet your body's nutritional requirement through the following:

- Keep your body well hydrated, drink at least 6-8 glasses of water a day.

- Consume a wide variety of nutritious foods

- Consume carbohydrate sources such as complex carbs (e.g. vegetables, fruits, whole grains, oatmeal etc.)

- Include essential fatty oils in your diet such as those that are high in omega fatty acid, buts, and avocado

- Suitable amount of protein for muscle repair

- Include adequate amount of minerals such as calcium, iron and zinc

- Choose to eat food that has huge amount of phytochemicals that will protect your heart against diseases of the heart, diabetes, stroke and some certain cancer

- And lastly, include fat-soluble and water-soluble vitamins

HEALTHY EATING FOR OLDER ADULTS

Babies, children, teens, young adults, older adults, pregnant women and as well as breastfeeding women all have different dietary requirement especially if you undergo stem cell therapy. The nutritional needs changes over time. As you reach this stage you will need to meet daily nutritional needs. Always aim to eat a well a balanced diet to keep your body function at its best.

For adults over 45 yrs. old, the recommendations are:

- Be pro-active, boost appetite and maintain the muscle mass

- Keep a regular workout, eat nutritiously

- Consume more nutrient dense foods such as eggs, low-fat dairy, fish, liver, nuts, meat, legumes, vegetables, whole grain and cereals.

- Spend time outdoor to get enough vitamin D to promote healthier bone

- Avoid foods that are high in sugar but low in nutrients e.g. cakes, pastries, soda

- Include high fiber foods in your diet for bowel health

- Avoid highly processed foods

- Avoid frozen pre-prepared meals

- Avoid high in sodium foods

- Drink adequate amount of water daily

Below is a sample 6-month nutrition plan based on 2000 calorie, you can choose from any in the Meal Plan A, B, and C:

MEAL PLAN A: (2000 CALORIES) RECOMMENDED FOR 1 WEEK BEFORE STEM CELL COLLECTION

Breakfast	Morning Snack	Lunch	Afternoon Snack	Dinner
1 ounce(s) grains 1 cup(s) dairy 1 ½ ounce(s) protein foods	1 cup(s) fruits ½ cup(s) dairy	2 ounce(s) grains 1 cup(s) vegetables 1 cup(s) dairy 2-ounce(s) protein foods	1 ounce grains ½ cup(s) vegetables	2 ounce(s) grains 1 cup(s) vegetables 1 cup(s) fruits 1 cup(s) dairy 2-ounce(s) protein foods

MEAL PLAN B: (2000 CALORIES) RECOMMENDED FOR THE FIRST WEEKS AFTER STEM CELL THERAPY

Breakfast	Morning Snack	Lunch	Afternoon Snack	Dinner
1 ounce(s) grains ½ cup(s) fruits ½ cup(s) dairy	1 ounce (s) grains 1 cup(s) fruits	2 ounce(s) grains 1 cup(s) vegetables ½ cup(s) fruits 1 cup(s) dairy 2 ½ ounce(s) protein foods	½ cup(s) vegetables ½ cup(s) dairy	2 ounce(s) grains 1 cup(s) vegetables 1 cup(s) dairy 3-ounce(s) protein foods

MEAL PLAN C: (2000 CALORIE PLAN) CONTINUED

MAITENENCE

Breakfast	Morning Snack	Lunch	Afternoon Snack	Dinner
1 cup(s) fruits ½ cup(s) dairy	1 ounce(s) grains 1 cup(s) dairy 1½ ounce(s) protein foods	2 ounce(s) grains 1 cup(s) vegetables 1 cup(s) dairy	1 ounce grains ½ cup(s) vegetables ½ cup(s) dairy 2-ounce(s) protein foods	2 ounce(s) grains 1 cup(s) vegetables 1 cup(s) fruits 2-ounce(s) protein foods

Reference: supertracker.usda.gov

Some important dietary supplements for stem cell therapy are beneficial by creating a healthier microenvironment causing stem cells to be stimulated to work/grow better, those are discussed below:

SPIRULINA

Did you know that the awesome benefits of spirulina have been proven centuries old with the highest nutritional value that a man can get? This amazing microalgae is a potent "superfood" and others even call it "a miracle from the sea". Spirulina grows in salty water and in freshwater as a type of blue-green algae or the bacteria known as "cyanobacterium". These special power food has a lot of benefits such as antioxidant, aids in lowering blood pressure, improve symptoms of certain allergies, improve muscle strength and helps in lowing cholesterol and triglycerides. This powerful antioxidant brings down the acidic environment in the body elevating alkaline levels beneficial to stem cells grow. It contains *phycocyanin* which has the ability to produce stem cells that has the ability to regenerate that your body needs.

RESVERATROL

It is known to be a natural compound which is commonly found in skin of red grapes (therefore in red wine), blueberries, peanuts and Japanese knotweed. This has powerful antioxidant properties that can protect our body from free radicals that destroy our cells. It can also protect our hart, lowers cholesterol and prevent blood clots that causes heart attacks and stroke. Resveratrol can also help in lowering blood sugar levels and considered antioxidant that can fight off some certain cancers. It is also considered an antiaging supplement. Resveratrol has the ability to help stem cells resist negative chemicals that's very important to promote health.

MELATONIN

This is a hormone that is produce in the body most particularly by our pineal gland. To regulate sleep and wake cycle. An individual who have trouble relieving or getting sleep have low levels of melatonin, which means they needed ample supply of this hormone. Melatonin supplement is recommended for those with sleeping disorders or overly stressed due to the side effects of drug related to lowering blood pressure, and can also be given for neurologic related patients. Melatonin also enhances skin wound healing with those having stem cell therapy.

WOBENZYM

Wobenzym supplement is a natural enzyme particular uses in digestive system to break down proteins, fruit enzymes such as bromelain that can found in pineapples and papain from papayas. This is widely used by many to help chronic pain, inflammation and for faster healing. Wobenzym also promotes stem cell multiplication and immune regulation therefore other benefits that wobenzym can give are for joint health, heart and circulatory health, surgery, injury recovery, and improve the immune system.

Food Recommendations & Substitutions For Individuals With Medical Conditions

DIABETES

Stem cells hold incredible potential as a source of insulin-producing cells. Take control of your diabetes. Choose high in fiber complex carbohydrates or also known as slow-release carbs and with limited refined carbohydrates. You don't have to eliminate sugar but more importantly, have it in moderation. Consume fat wisely and eat regularly at the required time to maintain your blood sugar levels.

High in glycemic index can spike your blood rapidly, while low in GI can lower blood sugar levels. Take a look at the following list of food guidelines:

Eat more of these:

- Fats from raw nuts, olive oils, fish oils, flax seeds, avocados

- Fruits and vegetables

- High fiber whole grain cereals and bread, legumes

- Shellfish, organic poultry meat

- High quality protein eggs, milk, cheese and

sugar-free yogurt

- Eat less/none of these:

- Trans fat (from deep-fried foods)

- Fast foods and sugary desserts

- White bread, refined pasta or rice

- Processed meat

- Low-fat products

HEART PROBLEMS (CAD, HYPERTENSION)

Researchers described that transplanted cells can survive and function in the body especially with those having heart diseases. Make sure to also keep your heart healthy with food choices can help reduce risk of heart disease and stroke. Choose healthy fats such as omega-3 fatty acids, olive oil, canola oil, avocado, nuts and seeds. Avoid trans-fat that is commonly found in processed foods. Avoid unhealthy fats, and be aware of the word "partially hydrogenated" written in the food label. Choose whole grain bread instead of white breads as an addition to your meal. Consume plenty of fruits and vegetables as it contains lots of fiber for easier digestion. Fish is a healthy option for healthy oils, such as salmon and mackerel. This aids in lowering your triglycerides. Beans and lentils are high in protein, low in fat with no cholesterol that's good for the heart. Diminish salt ingestion (table salt, as well as products with salt in within).

RHEUMATOID ARTHRITIS

RA or rheumatoid arthritis is usually treated with steroids. A profound healing activity by stem cell therapy is demonstrated on various forms of arthritis. It is believed that the cells, specifically the mesenchymal cells, produce anti-inflammatory agents does not suppress the immune response. Be sure to also include anti-inflammatory food such as omega-3 fatty acids that can be sourced out from cold-water fishes in your diet. This is proven to relieve joints pain and stiffness.

Examples are:

- Mackerel

- Salmon

- Trout

- Herring

- Tuna

To help reduce inflammation, also add more fiber to your diet by eating lots of vegetables, whole grains and fruit. Eating hamburgers, grilled chicken and other grilled meats that are linked to advanced glycation end products (AGEs) detected in the blood if an inflammation is present.

MULTIPLE SCLEROSIS

Promising results are shown in battle against MS or multiple sclerosis through the use of stem cell therapy. The transplant of stem cells can reboot the immune system of individuals with MS, which well-known responsible for damaging the spinal cord and brain function. A diet with low-fat, high fiber diet similar to those with cancer and heart problems can benefit individuals with multiple sclerosis. Eat more fruits, vegetables, grains, fish/seafood, and seeds instead of those artificially sweetened foods. Skip those saturated fats and soda/soft drinks that can irritate your bladder. Avoid diet sweeteners, such as aspartame usually an ingredient in all diet sodas and other diet foods. We suggest to use stevia whenever possible.

SYSTEMIC LUPUS ERYTHEMATOSUS

Stem cell treatment has a promising therapeutic tool for individuals with lupus. The amount of immune effects of these mesenchymal cells are beneficial combined with a healthy blend of food in your diet is all you need such as fresh vegetables, fruits, whole grains, protein and fish. Include more calcium rich foods to your diet as some treatment drugs can have side effect of thinning the bone, making the bones brittle.

Avoid alfalfa as these sprouts contain amino acid known as L-canavanine, it can wreck your immune system that will trigger any lupus symptoms such as muscle pain, fatigue and changes in blood results. Also avoid the so called nightshade vegetables as some people with lupus experience sensitivity to these vegetables. Examples are eggplant, potatoes, tomatoes and chili and bell peppers.

KIDNEY INSUFFICIENCY

Reducing the needs for dialysis, stem cell therapy for damaged kidneys are now being developed by experts. Also include foods that contain antioxidant can help neutralize free radical and protect from oxidation that makes more applicable choice for dialysis patients and people with chronic kidney disease.

Healthy food choices for the kidneys are:

- Red bell peppers are low in potassium a perfect reason for kidney diet.

- Cabbage are packed with phytochemicals, Vitamin K, vitamin C and fiber. Also a good source of Vit. B6 and folic acid with low in potassium.

- Cranberries protects you against bladder infection that prevent bacteria from sticking to the bladder wall. Also due to its antioxidant ability, this have been proven to protect against certain cancers.

- Strawberries are rich in phenols, a powerful antioxidant which help protect body cell structures to prevent oxidative damage.

- Raspberries contain *ellagic* acid. It's a phytonutrient that helps neutralize free radicals in the body to prevent cell damage.

CHRON'S DISEASE AND COLITIS

Stem cells can help repair damaged cells caused by inflammation through rebooting the immune system of individuals with Chron's disease and colitis but you should also begin combining it with a healthy diet. Experts believe that some patients can identify foods that will trigger gastrointestinal symptoms so by avoiding these foods that might trigger the disease symptoms, it's much better to stay away or avoid it. When Crohn's disease affects the small intestine, it will result to diarrhea and undernourishment. A person with such condition often suffer from anemia, low levels of folic acid, B12 and iron. It's important to follow a high-calorie, high -protein diet, as long as you emphasize eating a regular meal, with additional two to three snack each day.

Avoid these foods/drinks on your diet:

- Alcohol

- Caffeine

- Soda/soft drinks

- Dried beans (peas, legumes)

- Dried fruit

- Meat

- Refined sugar

- Spicy foods

PARKINSON'S DISEASE

Stem cells become beneficial to help grow dopamine-producing cells that can possibly treat Parkinson's through substituting all the damaged neural or nerve cells. It is also extremely beneficial for those with Parkinson's to eat a well-balanced and nutritious diet. Include high in fiber foods such as vegetables, peas, legumes, whole grains, and fresh fruits.

Make sure to choose foods that is low in saturated fat and

cholesterol, and limit the sugar intake. Moderately use of sodium is suggested. Drink 8 glasses of water every day. Usually doctors will suggest not to drink alcoholic beverages for any patient for general good health, but specially to your condition here as these may interfere on the effect of your medication.

ALZHEIMER'S DISEASE

A transplant new stems cells to reproduce damaged of neural or nerve cells is one solution for Alzheimer's disease. An individual with Alzheimer's disease or dementia also needs a proper nutrition to keep body strong and healthy. Lack of proper nutrition will aggravate or trigger behavioral problem and symptoms. Give them high in nutrients foods such as:

- Vegetables

- Fruits

- Whole grains

- Low-fat dairy

- Lean protein

Cut down refined sugars to their diet. (Avoid all kinds of sodas specially the labeled as "diet") But in later stage of Alzheimer's, loss of appetite is one big problem, you may add small amount of sugar to their food to increase appetite. Limit also their intake of sodium which can affect blood pressure. Instead, substitute it with herbs and spices.

EXAMPLE OF HEALTHY RECIPES

Beneficial for stem cell therapy because of high antioxidant, rich on vegetables, low saturated fats and protein content.

Spinach Quinoa Stuffed Peppers

Ingredients:

1 cup (168g) quinoa or rice, rinsed and drained

Scant 2 cups (460 ml) vegetable stock

4 large red, yellow or orange bell peppers, halved, seeds removed

½ cup (120g) salsa

1 tbsp. (4g) nutritional yeast

2 tsp cumin powder

1 ½ tsp chili powder

1 ½ tsp garlic powder

1 15-ounce (425g) cab black beans, drained

1 cup (168g) whole kernel corn, drained

1 ripe avocado for toppings (optional)

PROCEDURE:

Add quinoa and vegetable stock to a saucepan and bring to a boil over high heat. Once boiling, reduce heat, cover and simmer until all liquid is absorbed and quinoa if fluffy – about 20 minutes. Preheat oven to 375 °F and lightly grease a 9x13 baking dish or rimmed baking sheet. Brush halved peppers with a neutral, high heat oil, such as grape seed, avocado or refined coconut. Add cooked quinoa to a large mixing bowl and add remaining ingredients- salsa through corn. Mix thoroughly to combine then taste and adjust seasoning, adding salt. Pepper or more spices desired. Generously stuff halved peppers with quinoa mixture until all peppers are full, then cover the dish with foil. Bake for 30 minutes (covered), then removed foil. Increase heat to 400°F and bake for another 15 to 20 minutes or until peppers are soft and slightly golden brown. Serve with desired toppings. Enjoy!

Reference: minimalistbaker.com

Barley and Black Bean Salad

Ingredients:

1 cup uncooked quick-cooking pearl barley

1 (15-ounce) can, black beans, rinsed and drained

1-pint grape or cherry tomatoes, halved

½ cup finely chopped green bell pepper

½ cup (2 ounces) Monterey Jack cheese with jalapeno peppers, cut into ¼-inch cubes

1/3 cup lemon juice

2 tablespoons olive oil

1 teaspoon salt

¾ cup fresh cilantro leaves (optional)

1/8 teaspoon ground red pepper (optional)

PROCEDURE:

Cook barley according to package directions, omitting salt. Drain barley in a colander, and rinse with cold water until completely cooled.

Combine all ingredients and if desired, add cilantro and red pepper in a medium bowl. Add barley to black bean mixture. Toss gently and serve.

Reference: health.com

Roasted Loin of Pork with Caramelized Apples

Ingredients:

2 10-14 oz. (1/2 to ¾ lbs.) pork tenderloins

4 tbsp. fresh rosemary, chopped

4 tbsp. garlic, minced

4 tbsp. olive oil

1 tsp each salt and pepper

3 apples, peeled, cored and cut into wedges

PROCEDURE:

Mix rosemary, garlic, 3 tbsp. olive oil, salt and pepper together. Rub onto tenderloins. Preheat oven to 450°F. Place pork in a roasting pan and cook for 18 to 22 minutes or until a thermometer inserted into the middle of the tenderloin reads between 145 °F-155 °F. Remove from oven, cover loosely with foil and set aside to rest. Meanwhile, heat the remaining tbsp. of olive oil over high heat in a large sauté pan. Add the apple wedges and sauté until caramelized and golden. Slice the tenderloin and top with warm apples.

Reference: allergicliving.com

Oven-Poached Salmon Fillets

Ingredients:

1-pound salmon fillet, cut into 4 portions, skin removed (optional)

2 tbsps. Dry white wine

$\frac{1}{4}$ teaspoon salt

Freshly ground pepper, to taste (optional)

2 tbsps. Finely chopped shallot (1 medium)

Procedure:

Preheat oven to 425 °F. Coat a 9-inch glass pie pan or 8-inch glass baking dish with cooking spray. Place salmon, skin-side down, in the prepared pan. Sprinkle with wine. Season with salt and pepper, then sprinkle with shallots. Cover with foil and bake until salmon is opaque in the center and starting to flare, 15 to 25 minutes, depending on thickness. When salmon is ready, transfer to dinner plates. Spoon any liquid remaining in the pan over the salmon.

Reference: lifescript.com

GLOSSARY

- **Adult stem cells:** Non-embryonic, non-differentiated stem cells. These Stem cells can be found, among others tissues, in bone marrow, fat tissue, umbilical cord blood, etc. (Also identified according to differentiation capability: multipotent, totipotent and pluripotent). All the non-embryonic stem cells are considered adult stem cells.

- **Allogeneic:** Refers to the procedure where the donor is a different person from the receiver, reason why it is necessary to take care of tissue compatibility in order to avoid Graft-Versus-Host-Disease.

- **Autologous:** Refers to the procedure where the donor and receiver is the same person, reason why the compatibility is a match.

- **Bone marrow stem cells:** Adult stem cells obtained from bone marrow.

- **Cell therapy:** Refers to treatments based on regenerative medicine to repair damaged or destroyed tissue.

- **Cord blood stem cell:** Adult Stem Cell obtained from umbilical cord blood collected at time of birth. These UCB stem cells are on the move from the liver (where blood production takes place during the fetal life) to bone marrow (where blood production takes place after birth). It is commonly used for treatments of leukemia and other blood diseases on children, most cases have been on siblings.

- **Differentiation:** Process by which a stem cell acquires characteristics of a specialized cell line and becomes specific tissue cell.

- **Embryonic stem cell:** Stem Cell obtained from a fertilized egg (blastocyst) after a few days of fertilization and before cell differentiation. Embryonic Stem cells are Totipotent, which means they can differentiate into any kind of tissue cell of the fetus.

- **Good Manufacturing Practices (GMP):** GMP are quality standards. It guarantees products and processes are following and complying highest standards of quality and specifications of that product or process.

- **Hematopoietic stem cells:** Stem cells committed to blood cells (red cells, white cells, platelets).

- **HLA:** Human Leukocyte Antigen

- **Human Histocompatibility Test**: where immunological system markers of a person are determined. By this system our body recognizes own cells from foreign cells/tissue. HLA tests are meant to find tissue compatibility between people. When 6 markers are a match between two people, is said they have perfect compatibility. For transplants/treatments perfect match is required, but there are exceptions where 5/6 and up to 4/6 compatibility could be used acceptable depending on the patient, the disease and the source of stem cells being used.

- **hESC:** Human embryonic stem cell

- **Mesenchymal stem cell (Also known as stromal):** Group of bone marrow stem cells not committed to blood cell production. Mesenchymal stem cells are capable to multiply and different themselves in different types of cells.

- **Multipotent stem cell:** Stem cells that could differentiate into more than one type of cellular lines.

- **PGD:** Preimplantation genetic diagnosis, embryo-sampling technique where a single cell is removed from an eight-cell embryo. DNA is extracted to study whether the embryo is a disease carrier or not.

- **Plasticity:** Ability/flexibility of a stem cell to differentiate into other types of cell lines.

- **Pluripotent stem cell:** Are stem cells that could differentiate into almost any type of cellular lines.

- **Potentiality:** Is the capacity to differentiate into specific tissue cells. They are classified into Unipotent, Multipotent and Totipotent cells. This depends on the number of cell lines that they can differentiate into.

- **Progenitor stem cells (or Unipotent stem cell):** Are stem cells that could differentiate into a single type of cellular line. At the end of a long chain of cell division are "fully differentiated" cells, such as a liver cell or lung cell, which are permanently committed to specific functions of that tissue. It leads to the recovery of the tissue and they act as a repair system for the body. And they stick with the same organism throughout the life of it.

- **Protocol:** A set of actions, methods, and the observance of certain conventional rules, which are planned and structured for a procedure. Destined to standardize behavior in a specific situation.

- **Regenerative medicine:** Treatment where stem cells are induced to differentiate into specific cells type required to repair damaged or destroyed tissue.

- **Research Protocol:** A collection of information that describes the objectives, design, methodology and considerations taken into account in the implementation and organization of scientific research. Includes the analysis and interpretation of results. It also provides the background and reasons why such research is being carried out and defines the parameters under which it will measure its results.

- **Self renewable:** Refers to the ability to duplicate through several cycles of cellular division maintaining his state undifferentiated.

- **Stem Cells:** Primary cells able to multiply themselves (indefinitely) and to differentiate into cells of specific types.

- **Stem Cell CD34:** Hematopoietic Stem Cell with specific molecular structure showing a surface marking differentiator (CD refers to Cluster Differentiator and number 34 refers to type of marker showed by true stem cells).

- **Tissue engineering:** Refers to construction of new tissue based on stem cells. Tissues such as skin or cartilage could be produced outside the body and be transplanted later to the patient.

- **Totipotent stem cell:** Are stem cells that could differentiate into all body cell types and are able to form a viable complete organism. An example would be the cells of a fresh fertilized egg.

- **Unipotent:** Are stem cells that could differentiate into a single type of cellular line.

ABOUT DR. LUIS ROMERO

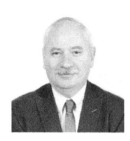

Dr. Luis Romero is an orthopedic and spine surgeon, an author, and published scientific researcher in the field of Stem Cell Therapy. Dr. Romero graduated from the Autonomous University of Guadalajara School of Medicine in 1980, with residency in Orthopedics and Traumatology at the hospital Magdalena de las Salinas which, at that time, was the most prestigious hospital in all of Latin America for this specialty.

In addition Dr. Romero complemented his career and education in different places such as Costa Rica; Los Angeles, San Diego, CA; Las Vegas, NV; Bordeaux, France and Buenos Aires, Argentina.

Dr. Romero has been practicing Orthopedic and Spine Surgery for more than 30 years in Tijuana, Mexico. He perfected the use of ozone for orthopedic problems, and developed a spinal cord injury research program. In reference to the field of Stem Cell Therapies, Dr. Romero started with Stem Cell Treatments for orthopedic injuries 25 years ago and has been researching it ever since. In 2009, Dr. Romero founded *ProgenCell*, a Stem Cell Treatment Center with and adjacent laboratory, to continue his research and to offer patients the opportunity and access to the latest technologies and most advanced techniques techniques in Regenerative Medicine.

ABOUT DR. JORGE GAVIÑO

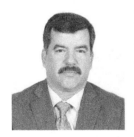 Dr. Jorge Gaviño is a passionate advocate of Stem Cell Treatment. He is a wellness champion and a visionary, and has a long and successful career alongside Dr. Luis Romero in the Stem Cell Therapies field. After 25 years as a physician to thousands of patients, Dr Gaviño merged his passion for health with his experience, and co-wrote with Dr. Luis Romero *A Patients Guide to Stem Cell Therapy*, with the purpose of educating and empowering millions of patients to take control of their health and learn.

After graduating from the University of Sinaloa, Dr. G, as his patients refer to him, did postgraduate studies in Tijuana (Hospital Angeles, Orthopaedics College & Universidad Autónoma de Baja California) and San Diego (University of California, San Diego School of Medicine & University of Arizona). He subsequently began working with Dr. Luis Romero as an associate surgeon, and in several hospitals in Tijuana. In addition, he started to immerse himself in the field of Stem Cell Therapies, attending different workshops and congresses. Dr. Gaviño was especially involved with Dr. Romero in his research on Stem Cell therapies for orthopedic conditions and injuries.

ABOUT THE TEAM

After several years of doing research together, Dr. Romero and Dr. Gaviño decided to establish a dedicated stem cell treatment center. While overcoming hurdles, *ProgenCell* was finally established in 2009. The Clinic focuses exclusively on stem cell treatments, treating patients from all over the world in orthopedic, neurological, immunological, ophthalmic and metabolic diseases. Dr. Gaviño and Dr. Romero created a multidisciplinary group of doctors and scientists that brought ProgenCell to what it is today.

Dr. Gaviño and Dr. Romero combined their many years of expertise and experience in stem cell therapies to write A Patients Guide to Stem Cell Therapy.

If you are interested in Stem cell treatments or want to know more about the subject, feel free to contact:
Dr. Luis Romero or Dr. Jorge Gaviño at ProgenCell

Phone: + 1 (888) 443-6235

Email: info@progencell.com

Websites:
www.patientsguidestemcelltherapy.org
www.progencell.com